Praise for

AN INTEGRAL FOUNDATION *for* ADDICTION TREATMENT

It is rare to find a thoughtful and scholarly blend of theoretical astuteness and clinical wisdom in a single book about addiction. The author accomplishes this goal by the skillful application of integral theory as a framework for understanding addiction and its treatment. *An Integral Foundation for Addiction Treatment* belongs on the shelf of every psychotherapist who treats addiction or is interested in the topic.

> —Philip J. Flores, Ph.D., ABPP, author of *Group Psychotherapy with Addicted Populations* (3rd ed.) and *Addiction as an Attachment Disorder*

An Integral Foundation for Addiction Treatment is a brilliant overview of a truly integral or comprehensive approach to what has now become a crisis level epidemic in America (and indeed, much of the world). The great difficulty, up to this point, is that there are several different existing approaches to addiction and its treatment, and unfortunately none of them have worked nearly as well as it was hoped they would. This has left the field facing an epidemic with no agreed upon solution.

Guy du Plessis takes one of the most comprehensive metatheories now in existence—that of Integral Metatheory—and shows how it can indeed integrate and synthesize virtually every major approach to addiction now existing. The immediate benefit of such a far-reaching approach is a direct application to actual cases of addiction itself, and wherever this has been tried so far, the results are astonishingly effective.

This book is for, first of all, either those who treat, or those who suffer from, a specific type of addiction. Guy walks us through a clear, easy to understand, step by step introduction to each of the major areas of addiction and its treatment, as well as demonstrates how this Integral approach draws together all of the hard-earned wisdom generated by each of the various schools of treatment—except now, all of this wisdom is brought to bear on each individual case, and not just a partial amount of it offered by any conventional, limited approach. And thus, second of all, this book is for anybody who simply wants to deepen their own self-understanding. To understand addiction in depth is to understand every major component of being human, because virtually every one of them is open to invasion by addictive dysfunction—and accordingly this means actually understanding oneself in general, top to bottom, and that is what this Integral approach offers (and thus among other things, it ties together Western forms of Growing Up with Eastern forms of Waking Up and therapeutic forms of Cleaning Up).

In short, this book is a thorough introduction to the major dimensions of your own being and awareness—many of which you very likely don't even know exist—and hence shows how you can bring a truly wise and compassionate understanding to "all of you." Highly recommended!

—Ken Wilber, Author of *Integral Psychology and A Brief History of Everything*

Integral Recovery pioneer, Guy du Plessis, single-handedly proves in this monumental volume that moving into and through addiction recovery—whether personally or professionally or both—does not require the sacrifice of one's faculties for critical thinking. To the contrary, in fact, what is implicit throughout Du Plessis' incredibly keen and nuanced analysis is a requirement that, when face-to-face with addiction's enslavement of so many, one must think both solidly and in-depth. In that spirit, Du Plessis provides us a carefully constructed, metatheoretical framework for both critiquing, and incorporating the best of, virtually every major perspective on both addiction and recovery.

What a relief, as but one example, to read so clear an articulation of how that which may rightly serve the recovering addict at one stage of his/her healing journey may be quite contraindicated, or at least be in need of significant supplementation, at a later stage. Sad to say, a not uncommon "one sizes fits all" mentality (Plato's part/whole error, which mistakes one correct "part" for the "whole" territory) pervades the world of addiction recovery. Hence, addicts in sincere search for truly individualized help turn away, and often perish, owing to the limitations of being forced to rely on any one given approach. The Persian poet, Rumi, puts it well: "What is honey to one is poison to another."

Du Plessis, in his thoroughly integral embrace, here at last provides all of us—recovering addicts and/or those who work with us—a roadmap sufficient to the complexity inherent in addiction . . . which really is to say, to the complexity inherent in being human. For anyone seeking a sound intellectual basis for navigating the real-life challenges at hand in addiction and recovery, there simply is no better place to begin than with Du Plessis' latest stroke of compassionate genius.

—Robert Weathers, Ph.D., California Southern University

For those interested in deepening their understanding of the treatment of addictive disorders, this book offers a wisdom and depth I have not encountered elsewhere in the literature. Du Plessis offers the reader a comprehensive and in-depth critique of the various theoretical models used in the treatment of addiction. He then offers us his own approach, one that integrates developmental, biological, social, and psychological frameworks necessary to the successful treatment of addictions. For recovery to be successful, he states that on-going attention to relapse prevention must occur, and this involves treating the whole person.

Toward that end Du Plessis has created a brilliant model that he calls an "Integrated Recovery Program". I would call it a comprehensive roadmap for those engaging in the treatment of addictions. His approach identifies six recovery dimensions, all of which are necessary components of a sustainable, long-term recovery process. The beauty and elegance of this model is that it provides a quantifiable and accountable recovery structure, where both client and therapist "plan and gage the complex recovery process". In addition, Du Plessis stresses the importance of attending to existential and spiritual underpinning that often drive the addict's search for meaning and purpose.

This book is must read for all clinicians, regardless of your clinical orientation or area of specialization.

—Patricia Gianotti, Psy.D., Academic Director of the Wayne Institute for Advanced Psychotherapy, and co-author of *Listening with Purpose*, and *Uncovering the Resilient Core*

Guy du Plessis' latest offering proves once again he is one of the leading minds in the field of addiction treatment in the world today. *An Integral Foundation for Addiction Treatment* is timely, concise and a welcome breath of fresh air to a field desperate for new perspectives. It is my hope that it becomes required reading for anyone attempting to fully understand the scourge of addiction in all its complexity.

—Adam Gorman, Psy.D., Licensed Clinical Psychologist

Guy du Plessis has written an important book. This book serves not only as a brilliant addition to the growing library of integral literature and thought, but also as a beam of light into the arcane and esoteric domain of academic literature about addiction and its treatment.

True to the prime dictum of integral theory and practice, Du Plessis speaks the language of his academic audience, but like a dancing Wu Li master he blurs the surface of things and leads us to clarity and depth—every deconstruction is a reconstruction, and every seeming dark cul-de-sac a new doorway that leads to the what and the why and the how and then the where to now and beyond, to the lofty mountain tops of our true human potential and capacities.

—John Dupuy, M.A., author of *Integral Recovery*

AN INTEGRAL
FOUNDATION
for ADDICTION
TREATMENT

AN INTEGRAL FOUNDATION *for* ADDICTION TREATMENT

Beyond the Biopsychosocial Model

GUY DU PLESSIS

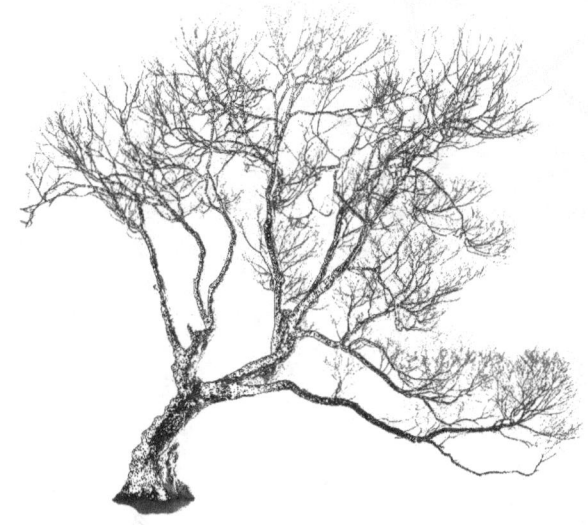

An Integral Foundation for Addiction Treatment: Beyond the Biopsychosocial Model

Copyright © 2018 by Integral Publishers

All rights reserved.

No part of this publication may be reproduced, stored in a retrieval system or transmitted, in any form or by any means—electronic, mechanical, photocopying, recording or otherwise—without prior written permission from the publisher.

For information about this title or to order other books and/or electronic media, contact the publisher:

> Integral Publishers, LLC
> 4845 E. 2nd Street
> Tucson, AZ 85711
> integralpublishers.com
> jcarlisle@integralpublishers.com
> 831-333-9200

ISBN: 978-1-4951-8778-0

Cover and Interior Design by Kathryn Lloyd, Integral Publishers, LLC: kathryn@integralpublishers.com

Printed in the United States of America

Freedom is the most ineradicable craving of human nature.
—JAN SMUTS

Dedicated to my daughter Coco

FOREWORD

Addiction studies is one of the most important areas of contemporary clinical and psychotherapeutic teaching and research. Although the treatment and researching of addiction is commonly, and mistakenly, seen as relevant for only a small segment of society, addiction and the human propensity for falling into the spiral of dependency are characteristics that lie at the heart of contemporary society. Wherever you might live in the world, addiction is present in your neighborhood in one form or another. Contrary to our conservative instincts, addiction is not a peripheral area of human experience. It is not something that afflicts only the marginal, the poor, the delinquent, or the weak. On the contrary, it lies at the center of our lives and at the center of the social structures through which we govern, educate, and entertain ourselves. Addiction is about nothing less than meaning and purpose in contemporary life.

Guy du Plessis rightly frames his approach to addiction studies within this broad context. He points out that substance abuse and addiction are among the most economically and socially destructive phenomena in contemporary societies across the world. However, the author also makes the case that the field is characterized by fragmented and disconnected understandings of the causes of addiction and how they should be treated. Theoretical fragmentation is not merely an unfortunate, peripheral issue here. Du Plessis argues that our theories not only filter and interpret reality, but also enact and shape the behaviors, social spaces, and structures that we design and build to bring about desired futures. If our theories are mistaken, reductive, or poorly designed, then so will be the interventions we make and the goals we aim for that result from those theories. This is one reason why poorly connected theory results in poorly connected health interventions.

One of the great powers of the human being is that we can shift and shape our environments to reproduce experiences that we find comfortable and pleasurable. This has great adaptive advantage in that we can build environments and design tools that make life easier, more amenable to flourishing as fleshy, sensing bodies in a world that is often perceived as insecure and threatening. The capacity to create environments also enables us to enjoy those things that we find rewarding and interesting, and to then enjoy them over and over again. We share this proclivity for repetitively sating our desires with all other creatures. Moths and humans are both drawn to "the light." Both are genetically predisposed to orientate their behavior with reference to that which is rewarding and attractive. Hence, we both can end up endlessly circling the light. The difference between us lies not so much in the strength of our attractions, but in the human capacity to create the attraction in the first place. Moths can't build lights but humans can. We spend a lot of our time manufacturing and acquiring objects and substances that give us pleasure and relief. Humans can and do spend whole lives, whole industries, and whole economies on inventing, designing, and building sources of attraction, pleasure, entertainment, and escape. Little wonder then that addiction and its treatment can be so complex and characterized by such a diverse range of diagnostic lenses and treatment approaches.

Du Plessis's book is a focused response to the pluralism of views and interventions that the treatment of addiction encompasses. Addiction is complex and engages all aspects of life and so needs a comprehensive and holistic approach to intervention. The author points out however, that, while eclectic and "holistic" approaches are commonly proposed, they lack coherency at a deep theoretical level and amount to little more than arbitrary and piecemeal groupings of interventions. He is interested in a more comprehensive conceptual understanding because this will have applied implications: "the more comprehensive our understanding, the more likely it is that we will be able to develop effective and sustainable treatment modalities."

Central to his endeavor of developing a more integrative framework for situating addiction models is the metatheory and metaphilosophy of Ken Wilber. Du Plessis utilizes many of the core elements of Wilberian integral theory and philosophy to argue for a pluralistic study of how addiction is conceptualized and enacted in addiction models and therapeutic practices. Addiction is complex and that very complexity creates the space for divergence in people's understanding, experience, and enactment of addiction.

The author applies the Wilberian integral approach (also called the framework, an abbreviated acronym for All Quadrants, All Levels, All Lines, All States, and All Types) with greater fidelity than is often the case. For example, moving beyond the standard four quadrants application of categorizing forms/theories of consciousness, behaviors, cultures, and social systems, Du Plessis applies all the five AQAL elements to theories of addiction and in so doing he nicely describes and co-locates a number of addiction perspectives to show how they might be applicable to particular domains of human behavior and experience.

The premise of the book is that integral theory, because of its metatheoretical background in recognizing and accommodating diverse theoretical positions, has great potential to serve as a conceptual philosophical framework and scaffolding for a more comprehensive understanding of addition and its treatment. While Du Plessis recognizes the benefits of pluralism and diversity, he also critiques contemporary addiction theories as being conceptually disjointed and fragmented. Even approaches attempting some form of holism such as the compound approach of the biopsychosocial model are still based on assumptions that reduce the cause of addiction to particular aspects of human identity and behavior. This fragmentation results in an overall ineffectiveness of treatment and so the impact of an initial fragmented and incoherent theoretical position ripples down through the diagnostic and treatment phases to result in poor outcomes for individuals.

In aiming for an integral model of addiction, Du Plessis sets his bar high. He says that a comprehensive integral foundation of addiction should be assessed by the following criteria. First, an integral model should connect the methodology, epistemology, and ontology of addiction. This is complex territory and Du Plessis makes an admirable attempt to identify some fundamental qualities of addiction theories and in so doing locate areas of strength and weakness in the current theoretical landscape. Second, an integral approach to addiction should include a developmental model that incorporates numerous growth-related etiological models. This is where the major strength lies in a Wilberian integral approach. The spectrum of physiology, emotion, psychology, and existential phases of development are ideally suited to exploring forms of addiction and Du Plessis weaves these elements of the human development perspective throughout his discussions on the many forms that addiction can take. Third, an integral approach should provide a framework that accommodates the plurality of models that theorize addiction from various perspectives. This is perhaps the strongest aspect of the author's work in that he provides rich detail on several very different models of addiction and recovery including the 12-Step model, existential psychotherapy, the compound approach of the biopsychosocial model, and social-environmental models. Fourth, integral models of addiction should be consistent with both the behavioral/empirical and experiential/phenomenological dimensions of living with addiction. A truly integrative perspective on addiction must take into account the experiences and feelings of the addict and their relationships and not only consider the objective realities of their condition. On this account, the book probably suffers from the lack of representative voices from people living with addiction and drug dependency. Nevertheless, there is the recognition that a conceptualization of the phenomenology of addiction is central to any adequate theoretical account of it. Finally, an integral model must be practical in that it can offer guidance for treatment and protocol development. In this regard, Du Plessis offers several interesting tools and protocols for assisting professionals in developing a more holistic and integrative approach to diagnosis and treatment. Although he states that: "It is up to the individual therapist to provide the details in the therapeutic encounter with his client," he offers a number of tools including "Integrated Recovery Indices," the "Integrated Recovery Wheel," and the "Integrated Recovery Planner" as resources for therapists. As to how well Du Plessis meets his stringent criteria, I will leave the reader to judge that.

In the final chapters, Du Plessis presents his integral model of addiction and its treatment. He aims firstly to provide "a new ontological and epistemological foundation for an understanding of addiction," and secondly, to apply this foundation to the treatment of addiction. His proposition of an "integrated recovery meta-therapy" (IRMt) is an original and innovative application of Wilberian metatheory to an area of huge social importance. IRMt is a metatheoretical framework to apply counseling, coaching, and psychotherapy techniques in a structured and integrated way to maximize the recovery and development of people living with substance abuse and addiction. Du Plessis offers a novel and interesting contribution to this important field; one that could make significant difference to the lives of people working to overcome addiction to find new meaning and purpose in their lives.

—MARK EDWARDS, Ph.D.
Assistant Professor, Jönköping University, Sweden, and
author of *Organizational Transformation for Sustainability:
An Integral Metatheory*

PREFACE

Attempting to understand and successfully treat addiction is a forbiddingly complex topic and endeavor. One of the reasons is that the scope of study and treatment of addiction spans nearly every discipline in the human sciences; it touches upon all aspects of what it means to be human. It is therefore understandable that researchers have mainly focused on studying isolated and abstracted features of this phenomenon in order to develop explanatory and treatment models. And those who have sought a more integrative understanding and treatment method have been faced with formidable conceptual and methodological challenges.

This book does not attempt to provide a better solution to the problem of addiction and the treatment thereof, nor does it present itself as a comprehensive overview of the topic. Its aim is simply to lay down the tentative outlines of a philosophical and conceptual foundation of addiction that may have the potential for theoretical integration and improving treatment outcomes.

As with any exploratory work, many of the ideas that are presented in this book are undeveloped and tentative, and require further investigation and critique. Furthermore, due to the vast scope of the book, and for sake of brevity, most of the topics discussed are presented as oversimplified and I was not able to do justice to its complexity.

My hope is that the integrative framework presented in this book may in some way enhance our understanding of addiction and its treatment, as well as inspire other researchers to contribute to the nascent field of integral addiction treatment and research.

I would like to express my gratitude to the following individuals who have either directly or indirectly contributed to the development of this book: Professor Vasi van der Venter, John Dupuy, Dr. Robert Weathers, Alwin Roux, Aristos Marinos, Spencer Hill, Marlien Wright, Ken Wilber, Lynwood Lord, Dr. Sean Esbjörn-Hargens, Dr. Adam Gorman, Debbie Fischer, Marie du Plessis, Lindsay du Plessis, Dr. Patricia Gianotti, Dr. Mark Edwards, Dr. Philip Flores, Dr. Mark Forman, Dr. Siebrecht Vanhooren, the staff at Integral Publishers, and to my beloved daughter Coco.

TABLE OF CONTENTS

Foreword *xiii*

Preface *xix*

Introduction *xxiii*

Chapter 1: What is Addiction? *1*

Chapter 2: Conceptual Chaos in Addiction Studies *29*

Chapter 3: Architectonic of an Integral Metatheory for Addiction *45*

Chapter 4: Integral Addiction Treatment *71*

Chapter 5: Integrated Recovery Meta-Therapy *95*

Conclusion *127*

References *129*

About the Author *147*

Index *149*

INTRODUCTION

If Dasein, as it were, sinks into an addiction then there is not merely an addiction present-at-hand, but the entire structure of care has been modified. Dasein has become blind, and puts all possibility into the service of the addiction. On the other hand, the urge 'to live' is something 'towards' which one is impelled, and it brings the impulsion along with it of its own accord. It is 'towards this at any price.' The urge seeks to crowd out other possibilities.
—M. HEIDEGGER (1962, P. 195)

Addiction, in its myriad forms, presents one of the foremost and mounting threats to the well-being of modern society. Addiction is the most ubiquitous form of mental health disorder in the United States and its burden on health care is so excessive and disproportionate as to constitute a medical and economic crisis (Kinney, 2003; Walters, 2007). The financial cost to society pales in significance in comparison to the daily human suffering that addiction causes.

As a consequence of the magnitude of this disorder, many scholars, institutions, and clinicians have sought to understand this complex phenomenon—as is evident in the abundance of etiological models of addiction in existence today. How a society views and understands addiction has great significance for addicted individuals seeking treatment. In premodern times, addiction was understood as possession by demons and seen as a moral aberration, and its consequent treatment was similarly archaic and punitive. It is only in the last 100 years that scientific theories and explanations for addiction have come into existence, and as a result, that treatment has become more effective (Alexander, 2008; DiClemente, 2003).

Although our explanation of addiction has become more sophisticated, there are still serious shortcomings in our understanding of it (DiClemente, 2003; Du Plessis, 2012b, 2013, 2014a; Hill, 2010). Furthermore, there is such a cornucopia of theories and models of addiction that for treatment providers and policymakers it has become exceedingly difficult to integrate this vast field of knowledge into effective treatment and prevention protocols (Du Plessis, 2012b, 2013).

The United States spends billions of dollars annually on the prevention and treatment of drug and alcohol abuse. However, the unfortunate reality is that most treatment programs have high levels of recidivism, with limited annual and lifetime coverage with low success rates (Alexander, 2008; Dawson, Grant, Stinson, & Chou, 2006; Hill, 2010). Furthermore, studies have shown that many existing rehabilitation programs may be no more successful than the spontaneous remission that occurs in the untreated population (Alexander, 2008, 2010). Despite the magnitude of addiction's negative consequences for individual and civic well-being, we have failed to make adequate progress in controlling or preventing the spread of addiction on a global level. Alexander (2010) lamented that a "century of scientific research has not produced a durable consensus on what addiction is, what causes it, and how it can be remedied" (p. 1).

Many scholars agree that two of the foremost problems in the field of addiction science and addiction treatment are definitional confusion (Shaffer, 1997; Shaffer et al., 2004; Vaillant, 1995; White, 1998) and the ineffectiveness of treatment (Alexander, 2010; Mill, 2010; Shaffer et al., 2004; White, 1998). Consequently, there are many that believe a paradigm shift is urgently needed, because there are such an abundance and diversity of addiction theories (Hill, 2010; Shaffer, 1997; Shaffer et al., 2004; Vaillant, 1995; White, 1998) that the field of addictionology is in "conceptual chaos."

What is currently taking place in the field of addictionology is what Ken Wilber (2003a) referred to as a "legitimation crisis"—a breakdown in the adequacy of a particular mode of translating and making sense of the world. Subsequently, the current move in addictionology is toward more integrative models of addiction that can take into account new data generated in addiction research: data which highlight the multidimensional, dynamic, and complex nature of the addictive process. Consequently, some scholars believe there is a need for a theory that provides a parsimonious and integrative explanation for all the existing empirical data—a theory that can incorporate and integrate the existing theories of addiction (DiClemente, 2003; Du Plessis, 2010, 2012b, 2013, 2014a; Hill, 2010; West, 2005).

In an attempt to find integration for all these divergent conceptions of addiction, there has been a movement toward holistic or compound models, of which the best known is the biopsychosocial (BPS) model (DiClemente, 2003; Griffiths, 2005; Levant, 2004; Shuttleworth, 2002; Wallace, 1993). This book highlights that compound models, such as the BPS model, have not accomplished the much-needed integration. Although the BPS model may be seen as approximating a comprehensive integrated approach, there are still considerable positivistic, ontological, and epistemological underpinnings and assumptions, namely, the abstractionist use of decontextualism, reductionism, and determinism, which hinder an authentic and comprehensive conceptual framework. The compound models do not provide a comprehensive metaframework to integrate these diverse explanatory perspectives or to explain multiple co-arising determinants. Current integrative models lack a metatheoretical foundation that adequately explains the simultaneous development, multicausality, and integration of the many factors in addiction (DiClemente, 2003; Hill, 2010). A truly comprehensive model of addiction should provide a metaparadigmatic integrative framework that highlights how various perspectives co-arise and link together, without having to reduce one perspective to another (Du Plessis, 2013, 2014a).

This book illustrates that addiction theories and definitions, like all scientific conceptions, begin with certain philosophical assumptions, which determine the nature of the concept and its trajectory (Bohman, 1993; Richardson, 2002), Consequently, addiction science, in its pursuit of etiological models, often shares a common ontological foundation with other scientific disciplines, regardless of its surface theories.

It has been argued that the development of an alternative ontological foundation could possibly lead to an improved understanding and treatment of addiction (Du Plessis, 2013, 2014b; Hill, 2010). The premise of the book is that integral theory has great potential to serve as a conceptual philosophical framework for a more comprehensive understanding of addiction and its treatment.

An adequate understanding of addiction has more than just epistemological and scientific value. It also has significant effects in the real world because the way that we understand addiction also determines the ways in which we treat it. Therefore, the more comprehensive our understanding, the more likely it is that we will be able to develop effective and sustainable treatment modalities.

Mark Forman (2010), a pioneer of integral psychotherapy, stated:

> Psychotherapists, perhaps more than any other group of professionals, are confronted with the full complexity of the human condition. So many factors—bibliographical, genetic, cultural, and social—come into play in the life of the client, mixing and interacting with largely unpredictable results. (p. 1)

This statement is particularly relevant when working with addicted populations because addiction is such a holistic disease—it leaves no area of the addict's life untouched. To successfully treat and understand addiction, all those affected areas must be treated, or at least acknowledged, for sustainable treatment. When working with addicts, therapists need a truly comprehensive and integrative therapeutic orientation to accomplish this goal. Joseph Califano (2008), author of *High Society*, echoed this sentiment:

> So, in research as in practice, this disease demands a holistic approach: combining brain-imaging discoveries, genetic markers, and new knowledge about dopamine, serotonin, and chemicals that effect brain receptors with all the psychological, emotional, and spiritual knowledge we can muster, to create a personal-environment antagonistic to drug use and alcohol abuse. (p. 79)

In order to treat the numerous areas affected by addiction and for recovery to be sustainable, many therapists working with addicted populations often recognize themselves as eclectic. Without a sound orientating framework this can result in syncretism, where therapists haphazardly pick techniques without any overall rationale and this consequently, results in syncretistic confusion (Corey, 2005). Many of the current holistic addiction treatment facilities are doing remarkable work, but on closer inspection of the philosophy behind these holistic approaches, albeit more holistic than more orthodox models, we find that they are merely stating the obvious: An integrative approach is better than a partial approach, without providing a truly holistic framework and method.

PURPOSE AND SCOPE

In an attempt to address the aforementioned problems (conceptual chaos and ineffective treatment) in the field of addiction studies and treatment, this book outlines an attempt at providing a new ontological and epistemological foundation for an understanding of addiction, and then applies this foundation to the treatment of addiction. This is done through the application of integral theory (Esbjörn-Hargens, 2006, 2009; Wilber, 2000, 2003a, 2003b, 2006) as a conceptual metatheoretical framework of addiction (hereafter referred to as an integral foundation of addiction or integral metatheory of addiction), as well as for a meta-therapeutic framework for therapists (integral meta-therapy) when working with addicted populations.[1]

With the ideas presented in this book, I hope to lay a tentative foundation for an integral metatheory of addiction. Such an integral metatheory of addiction should include several criteria. These are:

- It should provide an integrative conceptual etiological taxonomy that correlates methodology, epistemology, and ontology, and which as a framework is internally consistent.

---

1 The contents of chapter one to four of this book is an abridged version of my master's dissertation (Du Plessis, 2014b) as well as articles published in the *Journal of Integral Theory and Practice* (Du Plessis, 2010, 2012a, 2012b, 2014a), reprinted with permission. When relevant, I will reference the sections of the text that were originally printed in the *Journal of Integral Theory and Practice*, but will not reference the sections from my master's dissertation as this will unnecessarily clutter the text.

- It should include the developmental stages of addiction and account for observations of developmental models.
- It should provide a framework for understanding addiction as a multiple object on a continuum of ontological complexity. Furthermore, the framework should allow for various etiological models to address addiction at various degrees/stages of ontological complexity (*ontological depth*), and adequately explain and incorporate ontological pluralism (*ontological span*).
- It should be consistent with empirical observations of addiction made by clinicians and researchers, and with the phenomenological experience of addicts. Moreover, it must be relevant for treatment protocol development.

THEORETICAL ORIENTATION

The theoretical orientation of this book involves a (meta)conceptual/theoretical analysis of the existing theories of addiction. Since the data to be analyzed are theories and an existing metatheory, this type of conceptual/theoretical analysis is commonly known as metatheorizing. Mark Edwards (2010) said that metatheorizing "is a form of conceptual research that recognizes the validity of each theoretical perspective, while also discovering their limitations through accommodating them within some larger conceptual context" (p. 387).

Ritzer and Colomy identified four types of metatheorizing, signified by their particular aims (as cited in Edwards, 2010). Metatheorising can be used: (a) to understand existing theories, (b) to develop midrange theories, (c) to develop an overarching metatheory for a multiparadigm study of some field, and (d) to evaluate the conceptual adequacy and scope of other theories. The type of metatheorising that is primarily applied throughout this book is the third type: a multiparadigm study of some field (addiction).

Any researcher who attempts to metatheorize moves into murky waters. There are several difficulties facing any researcher using this theoretical orientation. Wallis (2010) expressed the opinion that although metatheorizing is a method that is used often, it is currently in a similar position to premodern science as a result of there neither being acknowledged formal methods in existence nor recognition by academia that it is an important form of research. Although there has been a resurgence of metatheorizing in recent years, traditional forms of scholarship still hold sway in this field. According to Wallis metatheorizing has as yet no formal research method, and there exists no thorough endeavour at appraisal of the (meta) theory itself. For several decades, Ritzer (1991) called for the institutional recognition and establishment of metatheorizing as a core academic activity. He said that metatheorists have been pursuing their endeavors in a "half-hidden and unarticulated way" (p. 318) and under increasing criticism from those who undervalue the role of integrative knowledge. He added, "Metatheorists often feel defensive about what they are doing, because they lack a sense of the field and institutional base from which to respond to the critics" (p. 318).

Edwards (2008a) wrote, "The 'data' of metatheory is not found within this empirical layer of sense-making but within the 'unit-theories' themselves (i.e., the individual theories that are the focus of study for metatheorists)" (p. 65). Metatheories do not focus on empirical events, but rather on the analysis of other theory.

Metatheory is grounded on the analysis of other theory in the same way that middle-range theory is grounded on empirical data. . . . Where theory takes empirical phenomena as its source of data, metatheory takes other theories as its "data" to be explored and analyzed. (Edwards, 2008a, p. 65)

Metatheory can simply be understood as referring to a type of super-theory built from overarching constructs that organize and subsume more local, discipline-specific theories and concepts. In short, whereas a theory within a discipline typically takes the world as data, metatheory typically takes other theories as data. Overton (2007) highlighted the metatheory approach:

Scientific metatheories transcend (i.e., 'meta') theories and methods in the sense that they define the context in which theoretical and methodological concepts are constructed. Theories and methods refer directly to the empirical world, while metatheories refer to the theories and methods themselves (p. 154).

Integral Metatheory

Edwards (2010) pointed to the difference between metatheory studies that are localized in character and metatheory that is distinctly integrative, which he referred to as "integral metatheory." Wallis (2010) described integral metatheorizing as integral in that it acknowledges the contributions and insights of a very wide range of theories, research programs, and cultural traditions. Integral metatheorising is characterized by its great scope, its openness to the diversity of scientific theory and sociocultural knowledge from all parts of the world, and by its use of other overarching approaches as metatheoretical resources. Edwards (2010) explained:

Research in any of these meta-studies activities becomes integrative [integral metatheory] when it: i) is consciously and explicitly performed within an appreciative context that can move across and within various disciplines, ii) adopts systematic research methods and principles, iii) uses, as conceptual resources, other integrative frameworks such as Wilber's AQAL, Bhaskars's meta-reality (Bhaskar, 2002b), Torbert's DAI (1999), Schumacher's system of knowledge (1977), Nicolescu's transdisciplinary studies or Galtung and Inayatullah's (1997) macrohistory, and iii) is characterized by its inclusiveness and emancipatory aims. (p. 225)

In short, an integrated metatheory is a metatheory that attempts conceptual integration, whereas an integral metatheory is a metatheory that attempts the same aim, but is specifically informed by integral theory. Edwards (2008a, 2008b) pointed out that a metatheoretical framework like the integral model has great value for scientific disciplines of all types because it has a potent adjudicative capacity for critical analysis.

One of the chief principles of integral theory is nonexclusion. This feature is of particular importance for the purposes of this book. This principle acknowledges that meaning-making is not sovereign to only one approach and methodology. Nonexclusion means that a metatheorist is indebted to the various paradigms of the many theories with which he or she works (Esbjörn-Hargens, 2009; Wilber, 2003a, 2003b). This principle is actually common in metatheory building. Lewis and Kelemen (2002) argued: "Multiparadigm research seeks to cultivate diverse representations, detailing the images highlighted by varied lenses. Applying the conventions prescribed by alternative paradigms, researchers develop contrasting or multi-sided accounts that may depict the ambiguity and complexity of organizational life" (p. 263). The principle of nonexclusion not only enables integral theory to perform metaparadigmatic integration of ontologically complex fields of study, but also to indicate the limits of the various paradigms that it integrates into a metaframework.

OUTLINE OF CHAPTERS

In Chapter 1, a brief overview of the most prominent etiological models of addiction are presented. The discussion is structured under the following headings: genetic/physiological models, social/environmental models, personality/intrapsychic models, coping/social learning models, conditioning/reinforcement behavioral models, compulsive/excessive behavior models, existential/spiritual, and altered states of consciousness models, and Twelve

Step programs. Finally, two approaches that have attempted to integrate addiction models are outlined, namely, the biopsychosocial model and the transtheoretical model.

In Chapter 2, the problems of definitional confusion and conceptual chaos in the field of addiction studies are discussed. As a result, many scholars agree that a paradigm shift is needed to provide conceptual integration. In this chapter, the fact that compound models have not accomplished the much-needed integration, due to the positivistic ontological, and epistemological underpinnings and assumptions which hinder an authentic and comprehensive conceptual framework, is highlighted. It is argued that the development of an alternative ontological foundation could possibly lead to an improved understanding and treatment of addiction, and it is proposed that integral theory could assist in the development of this much-needed foundation.

In Chapter 3, the architectonic for an integral foundation of addiction is presented, that is, a set of conceptual lenses that can explain being-addicted-in-the-world. Several critiques of integral theory that are necessary to consider in order to obtain a balanced view of the theory are also outlined.

In Chapter 4, the five elements of integral theory are explored as conceptual lenses for the development of an integral meta-therapy of addiction. Each of these elements are discussed in the context of its application when working with addicted populations.

In Chapter 5, I present, as an example of an integral meta-therapy, a succinct overview of my own model, integrated recovery meta-therapy, and provide a brief outline of its philosophical foundations and application.[2]

---

2 In the present study, the term *philosophical foundation* is used as a general term to accommodate both ontological and epistemological foundations.

CHAPTER 1

What is Addiction?

It is almost impossible for many young people to feel in any way useful in today's society. Why should we be so amazed that so many take drugs, and why should we interpret addiction as a regressive renunciation of the ego when the person making this choice is actually seeking a few moments of heroic identity? The archaic necessity of identifying both heroes and enemies become concentrated in the addict's creeping sensation of living a civil war between a minority faction, made up of angels of death, and a stronger majority of law-abiding citizens. The latter however seems to lack any identity of their own.
—LUIGI ZOJA (1989, PP. 15–16)

INTRODUCTION

In many respects, the development of reliable definitions, theories, and models of addiction is problematic. This is largely because the concept of addiction is abstract and does not have an objective reality or clear boundaries. Furthermore, addiction is defined socially and thus, views as to what the most apt definition is are varied. One cannot state categorically that some of the definitions are undoubtedly accurate and others inaccurate, but rather that some are more helpful than others, or that one is primarily accepted by experts (West, 2005).

A further problem is that theories in the field of addiction are rarely tested adequately in real-world settings because the dominant research methodology (based on a positivist paradigm) does not allow such testing. However, a good theory of addiction should explain a related set of observations, generate predictions that can be tested, and be parsimonious, comprehensible, coherent, and internally consistent. Finally, a good theory should not be contradicted by any observations (West, 2005).

Since 1914, the word *addiction* has been printed in the titles or abstracts of over 40,000 scholarly articles in the U.S. National Library of Medicine database. The term addiction can be traced back to Roman law. Addiction, however, is not a new phenomenon, and there are multiple examples throughout ancient Egyptian and Greek writings that clearly indicate their understanding of the problem. Interest was growing in the scientific study of addiction by the end of the 19th century. The *Society for the Study of Addiction* held their first meeting in 1884, but their scientific ambitions necessitated a formalization of a lay understanding of addiction. Early attempts at this formalization established addiction as a medical disease rather than framing it as a moral or spiritual issue (West, 2005; Alexander, 2008).

As knowledge on the subject grew, definitions across authoritative texts also evolved with time. Despite the progress, addiction always faced the same theme of a physiological adaptation to persistent drug use, and the absence of the drug leading to physiological dysfunction that results in often unpleasant or life-threatening withdrawal symptoms. An addict was someone that could only maintain normal physiological function by taking a drug. This concept of addiction is still given credence in the public perception as well as by certain researchers. They conjure up images of a heroin addict shivering with stomach cramps or the shaking hands of an alcoholic. This definition is attractive in many ways because it relies on the straightforward etiology and mechanism of action as a physiological problem. There is a physical problem that is observable and measurable, possibly even treatable (West, 2005; Alexander, 2008, 2010).

At present, addiction is generally understood as a syndrome characterized by impaired control over behavior, which leads to significant harm. This focus on harm is important because it has created widespread interest in addiction, which has led to large sums of public money being used to research, prevent, and treat it. In this paradigm, there is a complex collection of symptoms of addiction that go far beyond simply control. As a result, withdrawal symptoms, cravings, and tolerance are all included in the syndrome. Since withdrawal symptoms pose little social threat and are not the core issue, addiction needed a new way to be conceptualized. Even if withdrawal is dangerous to the individual, the symptoms are temporary and can be treated medically. On the contrary, the compulsion to use drugs or engage in dangerous behaviors is the primary long-term threat to both the well-being of addicts and those around them; this problem is much more difficult to solve with practicable and ethical interventions. Hence, from a social perspective it is much more deserving of attention (West, 2005; Alexander, 2008, 2010; Du Plessis, 2014a).

ETIOLOGICAL MODELS OF ADDICTION

In the following section, models and theories of addiction are explored. It should be noted that it is beyond the purpose of this chapter to provide an exhaustive discussion. The discussion is structured under the following headings: genetic/physiological models, social/environmental models, personality/intrapsychic models, coping/social learning models, conditioning/

reinforcement behavioral models, compulsive/excessive behavior models, existential/spiritual, and altered states of consciousness models, and Twelve Step programs. Finally, two approaches that have attempted to integrate addiction models are outlined, namely, the biopsychosocial model and the transtheoretical model.

Genetic/Physiological Models

The most substantial evidence concerning the role of genetics in addiction is derived from studies of alcohol dependence (Schuckit, 1980; Schuckit, Goodwin, & Winokur, 1972). Theorists have suggested that addiction runs in families and can be transmitted across generations. Twin studies suggest that a genetic transmission of alcoholism and chemical dependence is possible, and seem to support the importance of genetics as a contributing factor (Hesselbrock, Hesselbrock, & Epstein, 1999). What is, however, now becoming evident is that a genetic explanation for addiction will be polygenetic and complex, and will not lie in finding a single gene that can explain addiction (Begleiter & Porjesz, 1999; Blume, 2004; Gordis, 2000).

Historically, addiction and physical dependence were seen as synonymous. Addiction was traditionally characterized by increasing tolerance and the onset of physical withdrawal symptoms. Theorists of the genetic/physiological model of addiction have argued that the physiological aspects of tolerance and withdrawal are indicators that addictions are biological entities and medical problems. However, not all drugs and addictions produce withdrawal symptoms or create physiological dependence. Yet the physiological component of addiction remains an important one and there have been major advances in our understanding of the neurobiology of addiction (Roberts & Koob, 1997). Advanced neurobiological insight into addiction as having a physiological component and not constituting morally reprehensible behavior has led to it being understood within the medical model as a disease.

> The Disease Model of Addiction seeks to explain the development of addiction and individual differences in susceptibility to and recovery from it. It proposes that addiction fits the definition of a medical disorder. It involves an abnormality of structure or function in the CNS that results in impairment. (West, 2005, p. 76)

The disease model has played a significant role in shifting society's view of addiction from one of moral deviance to one that promotes treatment and understanding. Most neuroscientists studying addiction view it as a brain disease (Volkow, Fowler, & Wang, 2002). Addiction affects, among others, the mesolimbic system of the brain, the area where our instinctual drives and our ability to experience pleasure resides. This area contains the medial forebrain bundle, prevalently known as the pleasure pathway (Brick & Erickson, 1999). In addicts, the pleasure pathway of the brain is "hijacked" by the chronic use of drugs or compulsive addictive behavior. Owing to the consequent neurochemical dysfunction, addicts perceive the drug as a life-supporting necessity, much like breathing and nourishment (Brick & Ericson, 1999).

It seems clear, based on our understanding of the neurobiology of addiction, that physiological mechanisms and genetic factors potentially play a role in addiction; however, there are many concerns about assigning sole causality or priority to genetic/physiological factors. Although the genetic/physiological models are some of the most widely accepted models of addiction, they have also attracted much criticism (Blomqvist & Cameron, 2002; Moos, 2003). DiClemente (2003) stated that: "So many different individuals can become addicted to so many different types of substances or behaviors, biological or genetic differences do not explain all the cultural, situational, and intrapersonal differences among addicted individuals and addictive behaviors" (p. 11).

Social/Environmental Models

Many models of substance abuse have been criticized for not sufficiently emphasizing the role of social and contextual factors (Coppelo & Orford, 2002). In addition, many research studies have shown that some of the greatest risks of becoming addicted are related to the social factors to which a person is exposed (Sremac, 2010). The social/environmental perspective highlights the role of social influences, social policies, availability, peer pressure, and family systems on the development and maintenance of addiction (DiClemente, 2003; Johnson, 1980). Furthermore, an influence on etiological factors of addiction is the prevailing degree of attitudinal tolerance toward the practice in the individual's cultural, ethnic, and social class milieu. Research has pointed out that macroenvironmental influences also play a significant role in the initiation of addiction (Connors & Tarbox, 1985). For instance, since the breakdown of the apartheid system in the early 1990s and the concomitant relaxation of border management, South Africa has been targeted as a conduit country for the transportation of drugs as well as a new lucrative market for the sale of drugs (Myers & Parry, 2004). Poor law enforcement combined with sophisticated infrastructure and telecommunications systems have further compounded South Africa's vulnerability as a lucrative drug trafficking destination, resulting in the increased use of heroin, cocaine, and methamphetamine in the country (Parry, Pluddermann, & Myers, 2005).

Some supporters of the social/environmental models focus on the more intimate environment of family influences as a central etiological factor of addiction (Merikangas, Rounsaville, & Prusoff, 1992). They suggested that the onset of addiction is influenced by certain variables that emerge from dysfunctional family environments (Coleman, 1980; Kandel & Davies, 1992). These theorists emphasized that problematic family situations such as conflicted and broken marriages, difficulties with relationships, and the use of alcohol and other drugs by parents are important influences in the child's decision to experiment with drugs or continue addictive behaviour (Chassin, Patrick, Andrea, & Craig, 1996; Jessor & Jessor, 1977). Research has identified familial dynamics such as lack of parental support and ineffective parental control practices as high-risk factors for adolescent substance abuse (Hawkins, Catalano, & Miller, 1994).

It is clear that social/environmental models have relevance to our understanding of addictive behavior at a population level, but they often fail to explain individual initiation or cessation in any comprehensive manner (DiClemente, 2003).

Personality/Intrapsychic Models

Proponents of the personality/intrapsychic perspective link personality/intrapsychic dysfunction and inadequate psychological development to a predisposition toward addiction (Flores, 1997; Khantzian, 1999; Kohut, 1977; Levin, 1995; Ulman & Paul, 2006). For example, preexisting antisocial disorders, depression, low self-esteem, narcissistic disorders, hyperactivism, high novelty-seeking, and emotionality have been acknowledged to be possible precursors or predictors of later addiction (Jessor & Jessor, 1980; Kohut, 1977). This has led theorists to seek a pre-addiction psychological profile for people who have become addicted. However, a single addictive personality type has not been established in spite of commonly held beliefs that there is such a thing as an "addictive personality." Blume (2004) affirmed this when he said that "there are certain psychological disorders with specific clusters of symptoms that have a high co-occurrence with substance abuse and dependence .... but there is no single personality type for people with addictive behaviors" (p. 73).

A common explanation, from a psychoanalytic perspective, is to view the etiological and pathogenic origins of addiction as a narcissistic disturbance of self-experience (Khantzian, 1999; Meissner, 1980; Ulman & Paul, 2006; Wurmser, 1995). Kohut (1971, 1977) implied that there is an inverse relationship between an individual's early experiences of positive self-object responsiveness and their tendency to turn to addictive behavior as replacements for damaging relationships. Scholars who support the self-medication hypothesis believe that addicts often suffer from defects in their psychic structure owing to poor relationships early in life (Flores, 1997; Khantzian, Halliday, & McAuliffe, 1990; Levin, 1995). This leaves them prone to seeking external sources of gratification such as drugs, sex, food, and work in later life (Kohut, 1977). Khantzian (1999) declared:

> Substance abusers are predisposed to become dependent on drugs because they suffer with psychiatric disturbances and painful effect states. Their distress and suffering is the consequence of defects in ego and self-capacities which leave such people ill-equipped to regulate and modulate feelings, self-esteem, relationships and behavior. (p. 1)

The self-medication model of addictive disorders demonstrates that individuals are predisposed to addiction if they suffer from unpleasant affective states and psychiatric disorders, and that an addict's drug of choice is not decided randomly, but chosen for its particular effect because it helps with the specific problem(s) with which the person is struggling. Therefore, initiation of drug use and the choice of drug are based on the particular psychoactive effect sought by the individual (Khantzian 1999; West, 2005).

Ulman and Paul (2006), in their fantasy-based self-psychological model of addiction, showed that addiction is better conceptualized as a kind of self-hypnosis than a type of self-medication. They believe that an archaic form of narcissism, namely, megalomania is at the unconscious etiology of addiction. Like other forms of archaic narcissism, it could become developmentally arrested in the setting of a self–object milieu, which lacks empathy. In certain cases, such a developmental arrest may lead to addiction in later life. When using, addicts enter into a hypnoid or dissociated state involving an archaic fantasy of being a self as a megalomaniacal being endowed with a form of magical control over psychoactive agents (things and activities), and addicts then imagine that through possession of these agents they will undergo a metamorphosis or transmogrification into a radically new state of being.

Personality/intrapsychic approaches make a valuable contribution toward a better understanding of addiction; personality as well as intrapsychic factors appear to contribute to the development of addiction. However, as DiClemente (2003) argued, personality factors or deep-seated intrapersonal conflicts account for a possibly important, but relatively small part, of a comprehensive explanation needed for addiction.

Coping/Social Learning Models

Some theorists argue that addiction is often related to a person's inability to cope with stressful situations. They believe that, as a result of poor or inadequate coping mechanisms, addicts turn to addiction as an alternative coping mechanism for temporary relief and comfort. An individual's inability to cope with stress and negative emotions has been identified as an etiological factor in many theories of addiction. Therefore, the coping/social learning models relate addiction to inadequate coping skills, which result from certain personality deficits in the individual (Wills & Shiffman, 1985). According to DiClemente (2003), emotion-focused coping has been identified as a particularly important dimension from a coping model perspective. Some believe alcohol is addictive because of its capacity for tension reduction and its dampening of the stress response (Cappell & Greeley, 1987). Researchers have shown that increased drinking after rehabilitation treatment is associated with both skills deficits and the failure to use alternative coping responses (Marlatt & Gordon, 1985).

The social learning perspective emphasizes more than just deficits in coping skills; it emphasizes social cognition. Bandura's (1977, 1986) social cognitive theory focuses on cognitive expectancies, self-regulation, and vicarious learning as explanatory mechanisms for addiction. Moreover, this perspective highlights the role of peers and significant others as models. When advertisers use prominent public figures to promote a product, they are applying social influence principles.

Although coping and social learning perspectives have become popular in addictionology, generalized poor coping skills cannot be the only causal link to addiction. However, even if coping deficits do not sufficiently provide an etiological explanation, they certainly highlight an important consequence of addiction, namely, the narrowing of the addict's coping repertoire (Shiffman & Wills, 1985). The coping/social learning models attempt to understand addiction from several perspectives including a phenomenological mode of inquiry, a hermeneutical-interpretive perspective, a cultural anthropological perspective, and finally, an autopoiesis theory perspective (as do many of the cognitive sciences). Although the coping/social learning models do incorporate a multiperspectival understanding of addiction, they still chiefly focus on an individual's psychological processes.

Conditioning/Reinforcement Behavioral Models

The compulsive use of addictive substances and process addictions is governed by reinforcement principles. Addictive substances and behaviors deleteriously affect the pleasure centers of the brain (Blume, 2004). The stimulation of the pleasure center produces a euphoric experience that tends to positively reinforce addictive behavior. Reinforcement can be positive or negative. Reinforcement models focus on the direct effects of addictive behavior such as tolerance, withdrawal, and other physiological responses/rewards as well as more indirect effects described in the opponent process theory (Barrett, 1985; Solomon & Corbit, 1974). Positive reinforcement involves pleasurable consequences related to addictive behavior. Negative reinforcement, as described by the opponent process theory, occurs when a person is rewarded through substance-reducing withdrawal or emotional distress. Both positive and negative reinforcement play a part in the development and maintenance of the addictive process (Blume, 2004).

Some theorists have also suggested that Pavlovian conditioning is useful in understanding the addiction process. These individuals state that anticipatory drug-related behaviors can be linked to cues associated with the act of using the drug. Therefore, situational cues can elicit initial drug reactions and consequently, lead to the resumption of the addictive behaviour (Hinson, 1985). More contemporary classical conditioning approaches include cognition and physiological mechanisms in their repertoire of cues and responses (Adesso, 1985; Brown, 1993). This has led to an integration of conditioning and social learning perspectives (DiClemente, 2003).

Today there is significant evidence for the role of conditioning and reinforcement effects in the addictive process, and as with all of the previously mentioned models, it offers insight into the nature of addiction. However, conditioning/reinforcement behavioral models do not explain all initiation or successful cessation of addiction (Marlatt & Gordon, 1985). They predominantly attempt to understand addiction from a phenomenological mode of inquiry and by means of an autopoiesis theory perspective. These models tend to overemphasize a deterministic and behaviorist approach to addiction with disregard for many psychological factors, as well as providing an inadequate explanation from social and cultural perspectives.

Compulsive/Excessive Behavior Models

Some physiognomies of addiction, like the inability to successfully stop the behavior as well as its repetitive nature, have led theorists to link addiction with ritualistic compulsive behaviors. Theorists who link addiction to compulsive behaviors either come from an analytic or a biologically-based view. The analytic perspective views the compulsive component of addiction as reflecting deep-seated psychological conflict whereas the biologically-based view understands the compulsive behavior to be a result of biochemical imbalances reflected in irregular neurotransmitter levels in the brain. Adherents of the first view see treatment in terms of analysis whereas adherents of the latter explore psychoactive pharmacological treatments to bring the compulsive addictive behavior under control (DiClemente, 2003).

Some theorists view addiction as excessive appetite (Orford, 2000). Increasing appetite leads to excess and the developmental process of increasing attachment, which is similar to elements of the social learning model. Potentially addictive substances share not only the potential for excess, but also a similar process of leading to access. Both the compulsive and excessive behavior models share the notion that an addicted individual's behavior is out of control and that the addict is attempting to satisfy a psychological conflict or need (DiClemente, 2003).

Both the compulsive and excessive behavior models add some explanatory potential to some of the existing models. However, they do not highlight all the variables needed in order to adequately explain the etiology of addiction or why individuals continue to display addictive behavior.

Existential/Spiritual and Altered States of Consciousness Models
Research has shown that an inverse relationship exists between spirituality and drug addiction, suggesting that spiritual involvement may act as a protective mechanism against developing an addiction and that a lack thereof can contribute toward developing an addiction (Laudet, Morgen, & White, 2006; Miller, 1997). Some theorists have suggested that addiction is a spiritual illness, a disorder resulting from a spiritual void in one's life or from a misguided search for connectedness (Miller, 1998). Therefore, addicts may be unconsciously pursuing the satisfaction of their spiritual needs through psychoactive substances or addictive behavior. In a letter to Bill Wilson, the cofounder of AA, Carl Jung (as cited in Kurtz & Ketcham, 2002) pointed out that he believed "alcohol was the equivalent, on a low level, of the spiritual thirst of our being for wholeness, expressed in medieval language: the union with God" (p. 113).

Many addicts state that they turned to drugs initially because of an existential void in their lives. Drugs instantly provided a new and often spectacular sense of meaning for them in an otherwise barren existence.[3] A sense

---

[3] An existential perspective of addiction also highlights possible non-pathological origins of addiction. I tentatively refer to this non-pathological perspective as the existential dissonance model of addiction. Virtually all theories of addiction begin with the premise that there is something wrong (pathological) with an individual, and substance abuse is an attempt to fix it (pun intended). The non-pathological model is based on the premise that in certain cases (not all) if genius, skill, or talent is not actualized or provided enough expression due to internal or external environmental factors, it can contribute as a significant risk factor to developing addictive disorders. For example, having an extraordinary musical talent in an environment where it is not nourished, becomes a risk factor for that individual, where for most people not having the opportunity for musical expression would not be a significant risk factor. This model will also attempt to explain why among the addicted populations there are so many intelligent, sensitive, and talented individuals. That is the real sadness of addiction; it often destroys the best of us. And like canaries in a coal mine—the most sensitive die first. Society often tends to see addicts as congenital, morally or emotionally inferior human beings. In many cases, I believe the exact opposite is true. Due to their otherworldly sensitivity they are often the most susceptible to the pathologies of their environment.

of meaning and purpose is closely related to hope. Empirical findings show that recovering addicts who have hope are better able to cope with life's crises (Sremac, 2010).

> The archetypal need to transcend one's present state at any cost, even when it entails the use of physically harmful substances, is especially strong in those who find themselves in a state of meaninglessness, lacking both a sense of identity and a precise societal role. In this sense, it seems right to see the behavior of a drug addict who announces, "I use drugs!" not only as an escape to some other world, but also as a naive and unconscious attempt at assuming an identity and role negatively defined by the current values of society. (Zoja, 1989, p. 15)

Some theorists believe that humans have an innate drive to seek altered states of consciousness (ASCs) because they encompass systemic natural neurophysiological processes involved with psychological integration of orholotrophic responses and reflect biologically-based structures of consciousness for producing holistic growth and integrative consciousness (Grof, 1980, 1992; Siegel, 1984; Weil, 1972). Winkelman (2001) expressed the view that addicts engage in a normal human motive to achieve ASCs, but in a self-destructive way because they are not provided the opportunity to learn "constructive alternative methods for experiencing non-ordinary consciousness" (p. 340). From this viewpoint, substance use is not understood as an intrinsic anomaly, but rather as a misguided yearning for the satisfaction of an inherent human need.

> Since contemporary Indo-European societies lack legitimate institutionalized procedures for accessing ASCs, they tend to be

sought and utilized in deleterious and self-destructive patterns—alcoholism, tobacco abuse and illicit substance dependence. Since ASC reflect underlying psychobiological structures and innate needs, when societies fail to provide legitimate procedures for accessing these conditions, they are sought through other means. (Winkelman, 2001, p. 340)

For a comprehensive understanding of addiction, the inclusion of existential/spiritual and ASC perspectives is essential, although addiction is too complex for its pathogenic origins to be reduced to these elements alone.

Twelve Step Programs

Twelve Step programs have such a central role in contemporary addiction treatment that it warrants a discussion within the context of this chapter. Although Twelve Step philosophy does not provide a clearly articulated etiological model of addiction, it nonetheless has many implicit assumptions. In order to provide insight into the etiological theory of Twelve Step programs, it may be useful to briefly discuss its origins and the ideological assumptions that inspired its methodology.

Twelve Step programs are considered by many to be the most effective treatment protocol in the treatment of addictions. Furthermore, "Alcoholics Anonymous has been called the most significant phenomenon in the history of ideas in the twentieth century" (Kurtz & Ketcham, 2002, p. 4). Although there has recently been significant critique against Twelve Step program methodology, there is substantial evidence that the Twelve Steps of Alcoholics Anonymous (AA) is an effective treatment modality and a vast body of research literature substantiates this claim. Research has shown that Twelve Step affiliation buffers stress significantly and therefore, leads to an enhanced quality in the recovering person's life (Laudet et al.,

2006). A longitudinal study found that AA affiliation and the application of AA-related coping skills were predictive of reduced substance abuse (Laffaye, McKellar, Ilgen, & Moos, 2008). The same study found a causal relationship with AA affiliation and self-efficacy, as well as changes in social network support and abstinence, thus, expanding existing literature that suggests the same relationships.

Flores (1997) expressed the opinion that Twelve Step meetings provide identification, support, and sharing of common concerns, which are powerful curative forces. Only recently have professionals understood the therapeutic value of groups. What AA intuitively realized, Yalom (1980) and others are only now taking advantage of. Peers are often more significant than professionals in producing behavioral change.

History of AA and the Twelve Steps

The official starting date of Alchoholics Anonymous was in 1935, but actually it originated much earlier with its founder William Griffith "Bill" Wilson. Wilson was a seemingly hopeless alcoholic who made and eventually lost fortunes on Wall Street. He tried a multitude of techniques to control his drinking and failed every time. In November 1934, at Wilson's fourth and final hospitalization—at the point of hopelessness and despair—he was visited by Ebby Thatcher, a "hopeless" alcoholic like him, who was sober. Ebby Thatcher revealed to Wilson that he got sober after joining the Oxford Group movement as a result of a recommendation by Rowland Hazard, who was treated by Carl Jung. Rowland had travelled to Zurich, Switzerland in 1931 to enter analysis with Jung, after trying virtually every then-known cure for alcoholism. Shortly after his return to the United States, he relapsed.

After his relapse, Rowland was told by Jung that he "was frankly hopeless as far as any further medical and psychiatric treatment was concerned" (as cited in Flores, 1997, p. 263). The only possible source of hope,

Jung suggested, might be a "spiritual or religious experience—in short a genuine conversion" (as cited in Flores, 1997, p. 263). Jung cautioned him "that while such had sometimes brought recovery to alcoholics, they were… comparatively rare" (as cited in Flores, 1997, p. 263). Only much later did Wilson realize the significance of the story. Ebby Thatcher also introduced him to the work of William James. Wilson shared this information with his doctor, William D. Silkworth. Through the influences of Jung, Silkworth, James, and Thatcher, a series of events were set in motion that would help to create the foundation of the AA program. It was Silkworth's influence that helped to lay the foundation of the disease concept.

On November 14, 1934, Wilson found himself in a hospital, being treated for a severe drinking spree. On this occasion, he had what is typically described in philosophical and religious literature as a mystical experience. Wilson said of this experience: "I now found myself in a new world of consciousness which was suffused by a Presence. One with the universe, a great peace stole over me" (as cited in Flores, 1997, p. 264). The day after Wilson's mystical experience, Ebby Thatcher gave him James's *The Varieties of Religious Experience*. Wilson poured over James's writing and this helped him to understand and contextualize his own mystical experience and provided valuable insight for the future development of the Twelve Steps.

> Spiritual experiences, James thought, could have objective reality, almost like gifts from the blue, they could transform people. Some were sudden brilliant illuminations; others came on very gradually. Some flowed out of religious channels; others did not. But nearly all had the great common denominators of pain, suffering, calamity. Complete hopelessness and deflation at depth were almost always required to make the recipient ready. The significance of all

this burst upon me. *Deflation at depth*—yes, that was *it*. Exactly that had happened to me. (Wilson, as cited in Flores, 1997, p. 265)

Kurtz (1979) went on to explain the historical significance that the above insight of Wilson had for the development of AA:

> This was the substance of what Wilson had come to understand; also important was the meaning he found inherent in it, for his moment was—taken together with his "spiritual experience"—the third of the four founding movements of Alcoholics Anonymous. One-half of the core idea—the necessity of spiritual conversion—had passed from Dr. Carl Jung to Rowland. Clothed in Oxford Group practice, it had given rise to its yet separate other half the simultaneous transmission of deflation and hope by "one alcoholic talking to another"—in the first meeting between Bill and Ebby. Now under the benign guidance of Dr. Silkworth, and the profound thought of William James, the two "halves joined in Wilsons's mind to form an as yet only implicitly realized whole." (p. 20–21)

Wilson intuitively realized that this "deflation at depth" was a crucial component of his recovery process. Consequently, surrender has become a cornerstone of AA's Twelve Steps to recovery. "One submits to the alien and becomes diminished through submission, one surrenders one's isolation to enter a large unit and enlarges one's life" (Wilson, as cited in Flores. 1997, p. 266).

Critique of Twelve Step Programs

There has been much criticism against the Twelve Step program and its effectiveness from many individuals and organizations. Flores (1997) expressed the following opinion:

> As far as many professionals are concerned, Alcoholics Anonymous is a much-maligned, beleaguered, and misunderstood organization. A great many of AA's critics who write disparagingly of the organization do so without the benefit of attending AA meetings or familiarizing themselves with its working on more than a passing, superficial, or purely analytical level. They fail to understand the subtleties of the AA program and often erroneously attribute qualities and characteristics to the organization that are one-dimensional and misleading and sometimes even border on slanderous. AA has been called by some a cult, a religion, ideological, unscientific, unempirical, and totalitarian. Its members are said to be coerced into regressive dependency that fosters servitude, compliance, and the surrendering of individual control to a higher power. Nothing could be further from the truth. Such a stance completely misses the point of AA. (p. 249)

One must keep in mind that the Twelve Steps is an injunctive paradigm—a set of social practices. To truly understand the nature of Twelve Steps, one has to follow the three strands of valid knowledge accumulation: injunction, apprehension, and confirmation/refutation. This is where the problem originates with much of the critique of AA: To refute or validate the claims of AA, we have to follow the injunction first. It has to be experienced before one can confirm or refute the validity of the practice.

Therefore, attempting to understand the Twelve Steps objectively, without a subjective perspective gained by following the injunctive practices, is misguided. Pragmatic philosopher John Dewey (1961) called this type of distal knowledge "spectator knowledge." Dewey believed that authentic knowledge is only derived from one's phenomenological experience of interaction in the world. Wilber (1995) echoed this:

> One of the great values of Thomas Kuhn's work (and that of the pragmatist before him, and in particular Heidegger's "analytic-pragmatic" side) was to draw attention to the importance of injunctions, or actual practices, in generating knowledge, and further, in generating the type of knowledge in a given world space. (p. 282)

This may be phrased more simply as follows: "The first strand of knowledge is never simply Look; it is Do this, then look" (Wilber, 1995, p. 282). Therefore, if you want to claim any real understanding of the Twelve Steps, then "do" it—experience it—according to the suggestions. Without the "do," all consequent interpretations (whether negative or positive) will necessarily be partial, and misguided.

In the next section, I will briefly explore the Twelve Step programs from a self psychology perspective, as this will help to further articulate the etiological assumptions underlying its method to recovery.

A Self Psychology Perspective of Twelve Step Programs

Self psychology can broadly be described as a generic label for any approach to psychology that makes the self the central concept of focus. Self psychology views addiction as a disorder of the self and understands narcissism, which is a common trait for addicted individuals, as "the problematic expression of the need for self-object responsiveness" (Flores, 1997, p. 292). Addiction can then be described as a misguided attempt at self-repair. Heinz Kohut (1971) understood narcissistic disorder to be a consequence of an injury of the self. Kohut suggested that individuals' early dysfunctional experiences with others (self-objects) create a potential for addiction in later life. Drug addiction, alcoholism, or any addictive behavior is then understood as a misguided substitute for these missing relationships.

Put simply, poor relationships in our early development may make us more prone to addiction in later life. Typically, addicts have unmet developmental needs and therefore, some are left with an injured, uncohesive, or fragmented self. This leaves them feeling empty and incomplete and is the "hole in the soul" of which addicts often speak. Because their internal resources were limited, they remain in constant need (object hunger) of having their self-regulating resources met externally. Since relationships were the source of their initial wounding, they feel that they cannot turn to others to have these needs met. As a result, they project this object hunger onto external sources like drugs, alcohol, sex, work, and so forth, all of which take on a regulating function while also constructing a false sense of self-sufficiency, sovereignty, and denial of the need for others.

I believe that in many cases the type of damage to the self determines what type of drug or addictive behavior an individual is attracted to. Kohut (as cited in Flores, 1997) wrote:

> The addict finally craves the drug because the drug seems to him to be capable of curing the central defect in his self. It becomes for him the substitute for a self-object which has failed him traumatically at a time when he should still have had the feeling of omnipotently controlling its responses in accordance with his needs, as if it were a part of himself. By ingesting the drug, he symbolically compels the mirroring self-object to sooth him, accept him. Or he symbolically compels the idealized self-object to submit to his merging into it and thus to his partaking in its magical power. In either case, the ingestion of the drug provides him with the self-esteem which he does not possess. Through the incorporation of the drug, he supplies for himself the feeling of being accepted and thus of being self-confident; or he creates the experience of being merged with

a source of power that gives him the feeling of being strong and worthwhile. And all these effects of the drug tend to increase his feeling of being alive, tend to increase his certainty that he exists in this world. (p. 187)

The perceptive reader may already begin to see why Twelve Step programs are so effective in the treatment of addiction. In recovery, individuals learn to have healthy interpersonal relationships "in which the needs for self-object responsiveness (mirroring, merger, and idealization) are satisfied in a gradual, gratifying way" (Flores, 1997, p. 292). Twelve Step programs accomplish the above in a variety of ways. They supply "a predictable and consistent holding environment that allows addicts and alcoholics to have their self-object needs met in a way that is not exploitive, destructive, or shameful" (Flores, 1997, p. 292). Because addicts have unmet developmental needs, they have very strong and often overpowering needs (object hunger) for human responsiveness that may feel insatiable. Addicts also feel ashamed of these needs. Through identifying with other addicts, they start to accept these previously unacceptable needs and realize they are not unique or alone. One recovering alcoholic expressed this after attending his first AA meeting: "I told everyone all these terrible, horrible, and shameful things about myself and instead of being disgusted with me, everyone gave me their phone number" (Flores, 1997, p. 292). In Twelve Step meetings, they begin to feel the responsiveness and gratification they missed for most of their lives.

> If Freud was right about the apparent libidinal autonomy of the drug addict, then drugs are *libidinally invested*. To get off drugs, or alcohol (major narcissistic crisis), the addict has to shift dependency to a person, an ideal, or to the procedure itself of the cure. (Ronell, 1993, p. 25)

As a holding environment, AA becomes a transitional object—a healthy dependency that provides enough separation to prevent depending too much on any single person until individuation and internalization are established. Gradually, alcoholics or addicts are able to give up the grandiose defences (narcissism) and false-self persona for a discovery of self (true self) as they really are. (Flores, 1997, pp. 292–293)

Through working a Twelve Step program, addicts' infantile ways of getting their needs met are progressively exchanged for more mature ways of establishing healthy and intimate human contact, and thereby, they are able to internalize more self-care.

Kohut (1971) believes that there are three types of transference disorders that addicts with narcissistic disorders may have: idealizing, mirror-hungry, or merger-prone. Twelve Step fellowships provide addicts with an idealized other such as a Twelve Step program and fellowship, and a goal that is practical and attainable. If addicts follow the suggestions of the fellowship, then they may get all the mirroring and confirmation they need. Twelve Step meetings are always accepting and open, and act as a "good-enough mother that serves as a transitional object until the principles of the program are internalized" (Flores, 1997, p. 296). Twelve Step fellowships, sponsors and other sober members act as idealized others with whom they can merge: "Merger with the idealized other serves as a container for the depleted self of the alcoholic" (Flores, 1997, p. 296). Flores (1997) added that:

AA works because once initiation into the program occurs, contact with others is sustained, and through continued interaction with others, alcoholics are able to alter the dysfunctional interpersonal style that up to now has dominated their life. Khantzain explains that only through this maintenance of contact with others can the disorders of the self be repaired. He identifies the four aspects of the disordered alcoholic as: (1) relation of emotions; (2) self-esteem or lack of healthy narcissism; (3) mutually satisfied relationships; and (4) self-care. He agrees with Kurtz that it is shame that makes the engagement and contact difficult, if not sometimes impossible, for many practicing alcoholics. (p. 293)

The Biopsychosocial Model

Dissatisfaction with the partial explanations proposed by the previously described single-factor models has prompted some theorists to propose an integration of these explanations (Donovan & Marlatt, 1998; Glantz & Pickens, 1992). By calling their model the "biopsychosocial model," they suggested the integration of biological, psychological, and sociological explanations that are crucial to understand addiction. This model endeavors to unify contending addiction theories into an integrated conceptual framework. According to this model, addictive behavior is, therefore, best understood as a complex disorder determined through the interaction of biological, cognitive, psychological, and sociocultural processes. Addiction "appears to be an interactive product of social learning in a situation involving physiological events as they are interpreted, labelled, and given meaning by the individual" (Donovan & Marlatt, 1998, p. 7). The biopsychosocial model argues for multiple causality in the accusation, maintenance, and termination of addictive behaviors.

Yet there are several researchers who feel that the biopsychosocial model is also inadequate in explaining addiction and that further integrative elements are needed to make this model's tripartite collection of factors functional. DiClemente (2003) stated that "although the proposal of an integrative model represents an important advance over more specific, single-factor models, proponents of the biopsychosocial approach have not explained how the integration of biological, psychological, sociological and behavioral components occur" (p. 18). He goes on to say that "without a pathway that can lead to real integration, the biopsychosocial model represents only semantic linking of terms or at best a partial integration" (p. 18). DiClemente added:

> The biopsychosocial model clearly supports the complexity of and interactive nature of the process of addiction and recovery. However, additional integrating elements are needed in order to make this tripartite collection of factors truly functional for explaining how individuals become addicted and how the process of recovery from addiction occurs. (p. 18)

Without an orienting framework that can explain how these various areas coenact and interlink, the biopsychosocial approach often represents merely a semantic linking of terms and exhibits limited integration.

Although the biopsychosocial model has not provided the field of addictionology with a truly comprehensive and integrative model, it was one of the first models to recognize the importance of treating the whole person and not merely the addiction. This has contributed greatly to the application of more holistic treatment protocols (Sremac, 2010). A comprehensive critique of the biopsychosocial model is provided in Chapter 2.

The Transtheoretical Model

In an attempt to find commonality amongst the diverse models of addiction and seek integrative elements, DiClemente and Prochaska (1998) proposed their transtheoretical model (TTM) of intentional behavior change. The TTM "attempts to bring together these divergent perspectives by focusing on how individuals change behaviour and by identifying key change dimensions involved in this process" (DiClemente, 2003, p. 19). The primary developer of TTM, DiClemente argued for this model by stating that "it is the personal pathway, and not simply the type of person or environment, that appears to be the best way to integrate and understand the multiple influences involved in the acquisitions and cessation of addictions" (p. 19).

The TTM proposes that the process of recovery from addictive behavior involves transition through stages described as the precontemplation, contemplation, preparation, action, and maintenance stages. Different processes are involved in the transition between these different stages, and individuals can move forward and backward through these stages of change (West, 2005). Proponents of this model believe a person's choices influence and are influenced by both personality and social forces, and that there is an interaction between the individual, and the risk and protective factors that influence the pathogenic origin or cessation of addiction. This process requires a personal journey through an intentional change process that is influenced at various points by a host of factors, as identified in the previously discussed explanatory models. "The stages of change, process of change, context of change, and markers of change identified in the TTM offer a way to integrate these diverse perspectives without losing the valid insights gained from each perspective" (DiClemente, 2003, p. 20).

Although this model indicates an integrative principle that is common to all the previous models and highlights the dynamic and developmental aspects of addiction, it does not seem to provide a metatheoretical framework that truly accommodates all the previous perspectives into an integrative framework. The TTM focuses predominantly on one dynamic integrating principle found in all the prominent addiction models, but does not provide the metaparadigmatic framework needed for a metatheory of addiction. The model has attracted substantial criticism; West (2005) is of the opinion that "reservations have emerged about the model, many of which have been well articulated" (p. 68). Yet the TTM has contributed greatly to our understanding of addiction and recovery as a dynamic process, by explaining it through a developmental-contextual framework. Furthermore, it has provided clinicians with a dynamic developmental framework to understand treatment resistance and ambivalence as well as to identify certain developmental markers indicative of positive change in recovery (Miller, 2006; Miller & Carroll, 2006; Miller & Rollnick, 2002).

CONCLUSION

In this chapter, the most prominent explanatory models of addiction were explored. It is clear that there appears to be very little consensus regarding the nature and etiopathogenesis of addiction. Furthermore, the integrative models have not yet been able to provide the sought-after integration.

In the next chapter, the conceptual chaos in addictionology and ineffectual treatment are discussed. Critiques of compound models are explored in more depth, with a special emphasis on the BPS model.

CHAPTER 2

Conceptual Chaos in Addiction Studies

A paradigm shift is urgently needed in the field of addiction because, while the institutions of global health have expended vast resources over the past couple of centuries to control addiction to drugs, alcohol, and hundreds of other habits and pursuits, the flood of addiction has continued to deepen and spread.
—BRUCE ALEXANDER (2010, P.1)

INTRODUCTION

Currently, addiction theories are so abundant and varied (Shaffer et al., 2004; Vaillant, 1995; White, 1998) that the field of addictionology was described by Howard Shaffer (as cited in Hill, 2010), the Director of the Harvard Medical School's Division on Addictions, as "[c]onceptual chaos…a crisis of concepts and explanatory categories in the addictions" (p. 3).

Many scholars agree on two of the foremost problems in addiction studies and treatment. The first is definitional confusion (Alexander, 2008, 2010; Hill, 2010; Shaffer et al., 2004; Vaillant, 1995; White, 1998) and the second is the ineffectiveness of treatment (Alexander, 2008, 2010; Hill, 2010; Shaffer et al., 2004; White, 1998). Alexander (2010) lamented the failure of the field of addictionology to bring forth adequate solutions to the problem of addiction. He provided an in-depth and scholarly study of the phenomenon of dislocation, which he called a "condition of human beings who have been shorn of their cultures and individual identities by the globalization of a 'free-market society' in which the needs of people are subordinated to the imperatives of markets and the economy" (p. 1). He believes that the "only real hope of controlling the flood of addiction comes from the social sciences, which are uniquely suited to replace society's worn-out formulas with a more productive paradigm" (p. 1).[4]

DiClemente (2003) pointed out that in an attempt to find integration for all these divergent conceptions of addiction, amid dissatisfaction with the fractional explanations proposed by the single-factor models, there has been a movement in the last 20 years toward holistic or compound models. Furthermore, it has been suggested that the low success rate for addiction treatment is because substance abuse programs apply partial and outdated treatment models (Du Plessis, 2010, 2012a, 2013; Jung, 2001; McPeak, Kennedy, & Gordon, 1991).

BEYOND THE BIOPSYCHOSOCIAL MODEL OF ADDICTION

The integrated or compound approach to addiction is an attempt to integrate the divergent and often conflicting philosophical foundations of the

---

4 Alexander (2008) presented a powerful critique against the prevailing view(s) of addiction in his book, *The Globalization of Addiction*. Moreover, he presented an alternative view of addiction that is congruent with the argument presented in this book.

biomedical, psychological, and sociological perspectives of human behavior (Graham, Young, Valach, & Wood, 2008; Levant, 2004; Pilgrim, 2002; Wallace, 1993).

Compound models are based on the premise that the interaction of a number of distinct factors is adequate for explaining the etiology and maintenance of addictive behavior (Batson, Brown, Zaballero, & Faulcon-Gary, 1992; Griffiths, 2005; Griffiths & Larkin, 2004; Shuttleworth, 2002; Wallace, 1985, 1993). Compound models of addiction have been known by a hodgepodge of names, for example, the biopsychosocial (BPS) model, the multicomponent model, the multicultural model, the integrated model, and the complex systems model (Hill, 2010). These models and others are indicative of the discontent with single-factor models (Gifford & Humphreys, 2006; Shuttleworth, 2002). The BPS model is the most widely recognized compound approach to addiction (Shuttleworth, 2002; Wallace, 1993). George Engel (1977), a New York psychiatrist, is credited with coining the term "biopsychosocial." Engel asserted:

> I contend that all medicine is in a crisis and, further, that medicine's crisis derives from the same basic fault as psychiatry's, namely, adherence to a model of disease no longer adequate for the scientific tasks and social responsibilities of either medicine or psychiatry... The boundaries between health and disease, between well and sick, are far from clear and never will be clear, for they are diffused by cultural, social, and psychological considerations. (p. 324)

Undoubtedly, this approach implies that no one isolated causal factor is responsible for addiction (Griffiths, 2005; Hill, 2010; Wallace, 1993). From the BPS perspective, addiction is better understood from a framework that locates underlying links, namely, the biological, psychological, and sociological, as the most vital antecedents in the establishment of addiction (Gifford & Humphreys, 2006). Although the BPS model approach could be viewed as approximating a comprehensive, integrated approach, there are still considerable positivistic, ontological, and epistemological underpinnings and assumptions, which hinder a comprehensive conceptual framework.

The BPS model does not provide an adequate integrative conceptual framework for the many antecedent variables that it acknowledges and provides semantic linking at best (Alexander, 2008; DiClemente, 2003; Hill, 2010). Hill (2010) said: "Notwithstanding the apparent willingness to acknowledge multiple factors in addiction; simply classifying a model by a compound expression, as we will discover, does not automatically eliminate fundamentally abstractionists' [natural scientific or positivist] assumptions" (p. 107). Hill qualified the above statement by indicating the "abstractionist use of de-contextualism, reductionism, and determinism in the biopsychosocial model of addiction" (p. 107).

Ontological foundation

In philosophy, the term ontology is often used within the context of metaphysics, and refers to what exists or what can exist in the world. Epistemology refers to the nature of human knowledge and understanding that can be obtained through various types of investigation (Slife, 2005). Ontological and epistemological questions often are concerned with what is referred to as a person's Weltanschauung, or worldview.

Philosophers and theoretical psychologists point out that all theories have ontological and epistemological ancestry or foundational assumptions, whether implicitly or explicitly stated (Bishop, 2007; Polkinghorn, 2004; Slife, 2005). Consequently, conceptions of addiction, like conceptions in any science, are based on certain philosophical assumptions, which influence the trajectory of the development of the concept (Bohman, 1993; Richardson,

2002). In addiction science, these initial assumptions often go unnoticed and consequently, are uncontested once treatment methodologies are employed and made the objects of research (Hill, 2010).

Ribes-Inesta (2003), for example, commented "psychologists have paid little attention to the nature of concepts they use, to the assumptions that underlie their theories, and the ways such concepts are applied in the study of behavior" (p. 147). Within the field of psychology there exists various ontological worldviews and hidden assumptions. Therefore, theories about and definitions of addiction and treatment methodologies may in the same manner have been influenced by ontological assumptions, which often remain implicit (Hill, 2010).

Hill (2010) argued that there are certain (often unrecognized) ontological assumptions made by those who study addiction (or any human behavior), and he pointed out that most of these assumptions are abstractionist or positivist, which he said were problematic; as a better alternative, he suggested a "relational ontological foundation." His argument rests on the premise that if most addiction theories share the same ontological and epistemological foundation—all of which have not provided an adequate explanation for addiction—then perhaps an alternative ontological philosophy will bring forth unique insights. A brief evaluation of Hill's argument reveals the foundational shortcomings of most (if not all) contemporary compound models.

According to Hill (2010), most of the myriad (and often conflicting) etiological models of addiction actually share a similar ontological foundation. He further suggested a solution to the conceptual chaos surrounding addiction studies. He summed up his main premise by saying that:

> First, I will suggest that the conceptual confusion surrounding addiction is more apparent than real, that there is in fact, a shared unity at the ontological level. Second, if it is true

that most conceptions share a similar ontological basis, then perhaps an alternative ontological viewpoint could offer a fresh approach to addiction and conceivably lead to greater treatment effectiveness. (p. 5)

According to Hill (2010) there are the two major ontological categories or foundations applied in the social sciences to understand human behavior: ontological abstractionism and ontological relationality (Bishop, 2007; Slife, 2005). Since addiction is often described in terms of human behavior (Brodie & Redfield, 2002; Flores, 1997), he investigated how these two ontological foundations underpin many studies of addiction. Hill discussed the ontological assumptions of the disease model, the life-process model, and the compound model; most researchers have agreed that these three generalized frameworks include the full spectrum of etiological theories (Campbell, 1996; Shaffer et al., 2004). His evaluation of these three broad classes of addiction models reveals a domination of an abstractionist or positivistic ontology.

An overview is provided of the positivistic or abstractionist ontology, which as Hill (2010) astutely indicated, underlies most addiction models including the biopsychosocial model. Thereafter, a synopsis follows of Hill's suggestion of a relational ontology as an alternative foundation for addiction studies.

Ontological abstractionism of addiction

Abstractionism is a way of viewing the world that identifies or considers all ontological reality as independent and isolated (Slife & Richardson, 2008). Abstractionism attempts, therefore, to isolate events from the context in which they occur, in order to obtain an unbiased understanding. "The key idea [behind abstractionism] is to isolate the properties in question from the rest of the environment and analyze them in as context-free a manner as possible" (Bishop, 2007, p. 114).

Ontological abstractionism, therefore, "assume[s] that all things, including the self, are the most real and best understood when they are separated from the situations in which they occur" (Slife, as cited in Hill, 2010, p. 15). This isolation gives rise to "law-like connections between causes and effects" (Bishop, 2007, p. 115). According to Hill (2010), "Addiction concepts from the abstractionist perspective would therefore only accept a contextless and individualist approach as the most fundamental way in which to understand and treat the disorder" (p. 15). An abstractionist ontology of addiction is to be "found in self-contained or isolatable factors considered to be basically unchanged and or at least similar from context to context" (p. 16).

The assumption of unchangeableness implies that addiction within an individual remains basically unchanged from context to context. Many contemporary models of addiction underscore this abstractionist notion of unchangeableness (Flores, 1997; White, 1998). For example, the disease model views addiction as residing within the individual, and continues to live on within the individual even after many years of abstinence (Flores, 1997; Menninger, 1938; Vaillant, 1995). In short, addiction from the abstractionist position is viewed as "consistent regardless of the context in which the individual is found" (Hill, 2010, p. 16).

Ontological relationality

In contrast to this abstractionist ontology, Hill (2010) proposed a relational ontology as a foundation for understanding addiction: "Ontological relationality, by contrast, is a philosophy that asserts individuals and their behaviors can only be understood in relation to the contexts in which the individual exists or the behavior occurs" (p. 16).

Addiction from a relational perspective would likewise not only value the similarities evident from context to context, but would also acknowledge the influence of contexts and relationships on the most basic meanings of addiction. Furthermore, factors associated with addiction would be conceived of not as self-contained or autonomous but as inter-related and *mutually constitutive* of other pertinent factors. Mutually constitutive refers to how each factor never exists as a self-contained entity but only in relationship to other factors. Pertinent factors are thus necessary for addiction to occur but not sufficient in and of themselves to account for the disorder. This suggests that factors of addiction, e.g., genetics, environment, and the contexts in which they occur, are not sufficient or "the cause" in and of themselves because they are not self-contained and do not remain fixed from context to context. (Hill, 2010, p. 17)

Hill (2010) implied that the concept of addiction is subject to context. Essentially, "a relational approach would view contexts and relationships as indispensable when trying to comprehend, conceptualize, and therefore treat addiction" (p. 17).

I agree with Hill (2010) that in order to arrive at a satisfactory explanation of addiction there needs to be a fundamental departure from conventional ontology. However, I am critical of the idea that the potential solution is to be found in his suggested relational ontology. This critique will be discussed in a subsequent section.

The Two-Fold Problem of the Biopsychosocial Model

On the surface, the BPS model of addiction seems to offer an integrative approach. As its name suggests, the researchers who adhere to this approach are often uncomfortable with the theoretical shortfalls of single-construct approaches (Levant, 2004; Wallace, 1993). Griffiths (2005) echoed this: "Research and clinical interventions [for addiction] are best served by a biopsychosocial approach that incorporates the best strands of contemporary psychology, biology, and sociology" (p. 195).

When undertaking an analysis of the BPS's ontological foundations, Hill's (2010) critique of the BPS model is two-fold. He described the BPS model's shortcomings in terms of (a) the separation of factors and (b) the prioritization of factors.

Separation of factors

Griffiths's (2005) postulation that "interventions are best served" by the "best strands" (p. 195) of biological, psychological, and sociological units implies that they are also best conceptualized as separate or "self-contained individualities" (Slife, 2005, p. 3).

> Consequently, the biological context is decontextualized from the psychological context, etc. That is to say biology is abstracted from or does not serve as a context for the psychological. . . . Thus, the phenomenon of addiction as a "whole", according to the BPS model, is most meaningful when thought of as decontextualized or self-contained "strands." (Hill, 2010, p. 536)

Engel (1980) confirmed the existence of abstractions, by means of self-contained entities, in the BPS model. He is of the opinion that:

> Each system [within the BPS framework] as a whole has its own unique characteristics and dynamics. . . . The designation "system" bespeaks the existence of a stable configuration in time and space. . . . Stable configuration also implies the

existence of boundaries between organized systems. . . . Each level in the hierarchy represents an organized dynamic whole, a system of sufficient persistence and identity to justify being named. Its name reflects its distinctive properties and characteristics. (pp. 536–538)

Here the BPS model is regarded as a hierarchical system with "its own unique characteristics and dynamics . . . a stable configuration in time and space [which also] implies the existence of boundaries" (Engel, 1980, pp. 536–538). Therefore, each of the systems is abstracted from the other. Such a viewpoint naturally diminishes the whole of a disease to an assortment of "table configurations in time and space" (Engel, 1980, p. 536).

When we apply Engle's viewpoint of disease to addiction it can be reduced to a "stable configuration [with] boundaries between organized systems" (p. 536). Separation of factors is thus assured because each of these self-contained factors demonstrate "sufficient persistence and identity to justify being named" (p. 536).

Hill (2010) rightly pointed out when there are, albeit implicitly, a separation of factors present within the conceptual scaffolding of the BPS model, it cannot be called a truly integrated approach, and it does not adequately explain the coexisting and co-arising of the various factors.

Prioritizing of factors

In the previous section, the BPS model's supposition that "separating [the] factors of addiction" is the best way to "conceptualize the disorder" (Hill, 2010, p. 112) was highlighted. As a result of these factors being separated, it is tempting for most researchers to prioritize certain factors. Many leading supporters of the BPS model emphasize the role of neurobiology in the etiology and maintenance of diseases such as addiction.

In his presidential address for the journal *Psychosomatic Medicine*, Williams (1994) wrote, "My major message is that optimal growth in our understanding of how biopsychosocial factors interact in the etiology and course of human disease will come only if our research incorporates theories and techniques from neurobiology and cellular and molecular biology" (p. 308). Further highlighting Williams's (1994) prioritization of biological factors, he believes that the serotonin deficiency hypothesis is a fundamental explanation for early death due to "increased alcohol consumption" (p. 311). Williams (1994) asserted:

> Rather than saying that a hostile personality trait somehow "causes" the clustering of the characteristics making up the hostility syndrome, I am proposing that all the characteristics [including smoking, eating, and alcohol use] . . . could be the result of a single underlying neurological condition [or] mechanism: deficient central nervous system (CNS) serotonergic function. . . . Low CNS serotonin function has effects on biology and behavior that could be responsible for both the biobehavioral traits and consequent high rates of disease and death that have been found associated with high hostility. . . . There is very convincing and extensive evidence that weak brain serotonin function contributes to increased alcohol consumption. (pp. 310-311)

Locating "a single neurological condition [or] mechanism" as the primary causal factor of a variety of diseases illustrates the reductionist conception to attribute "the material of the body (biology) alone for explaining our minds and behaviors" (Slife & Hopkins, 2005, p. 2). In referring to Williams's comments, Hill (2010) pointed out "three ways in which abstractions [reductionist/natural scientific foundations] underlie this particular approach to addiction" (p. 103). Firstly, death is reduced to "coronary disease . . . and increased alcohol consumption," which is reduced to hostility, which is reduced to "low serotonin function . . . [in the] CNS" (p. 113). With low serotonin function being the final reduction, there is clearly a prioritization of neurological structures.

Secondly, Hill (2010) pointed out that the primacy and supremacy of neurological mechanisms are implicit by situating "a single underlying condition," (Williams, 1994, p. 311) that is, serotonin deficiency as the primary underlying causal link to which disease states such as increased alcohol consumption" are attributed. Thus, the underlying condition" of "low serotonin function" (Williams, 1994, p. 311) is established as the principal feature of both "biology and behaviour", which, in turn, determines to a great extent "increased alcohol consumption" (Williams, 1994, p. 311).

Finally, Hill (2010) pointed out that Williams labels human behaviors as "those that may otherwise be listed under a psychosocial heading, e.g. increased smoking, increased eating, and increased alcohol use. . . . [as] "biobehavioral traits" (pp. 114–115), even further distancing these factors from their overall context. The above is an example of how "the central proposition of neuroscience is that the mechanisms of biology are sufficient to explain the human mind and behaviors [such as addiction] . . . whereby other, nonmaterial and nonbiological are viewed as less than fundamental or unimportant" (Slife & Hopkins, 2005, pp. 2–3).

Although some researchers have established a relationship between biological factors, heritable personality traits, and psychosocial factors, the "relationship is ontologically weak due to the reduction of factors to the self-contained properties of each" (Hill, 2010, p. 116). Moreover, biology is so profoundly decontextualized or self-contained that the interaction of the ontologically less basic psychosocial factors does not fundamentally change the essence of biology, but only amplifies its self-contained properties. In contrast, Hill (2010) pointed out the value of a relational approach:

> By comparison, relationality would assume that biological and psychosocial factors share a mutually constitutive relationship with one another. They are each necessary conditions for the phenomenon being explained; no single condition is more or less necessary than—or more or less in control of—any of the others. (p. 124)

Therefore, biology—as a self-contained entity—is not "amplified by [self-contained] psychosocial factors," but rather each entity serves to give meaning and identity to one another (Paris, as cited in Hill, 2010, p. 117).

INEFFECTUAL TREATMENT

Considering the variety of treatment options, treatment efficacy for addiction is ostensibly low (Alexander, 2008; Dawson et al., 2006). Hill (2010) indicated that "large population analyses indicate relapse rates following treatment of alcohol dependence disorders to be between 70% and 90% and success in treating illicit drugs is even more discouraging, with recidivism rates exceeding 90% in many demographics" (p. 4). White (1998), the author of *Slaying the Dragon: The History of Addiction Treatment and Recovery in America*, echoed the above sentiment: "With our two centuries of accumulated knowledge and the best available treatments, there still exist[s] no cure for addiction, and only a minority of addicted clients achieves sustained recovery following our intervention in their lives" (p. 342).

It is important to note that the ineffectiveness of the treatment is not due to a lack of attention or lack of genuine exertion by concerned groups (Flores, 1997; Ray & Ksir, 2004; White, 1998). Progress in public health in such issues as sanitation, epidemiology, emergency medicine, and drug therapies has instilled hope that many diseases could also be treated effectively (Hoffman & Goldfrank, 1990; O'Brien, 1997). Unfortunately, the progress in public health has not been duplicated with regard to the treatment of addiction (Fields, 1998; Ray & Ksir, 2004; White, 1998).

CONCLUSION

In this chapter it was shown that the compound models of addiction such as the BPS model are built on a positivistic foundation, which by default provides a less than adequate conceptual framework for complex human behavior-in-the-world, such as addiction.[5] I agree with Hill (2010) that a fundamental departure from conventional ontology is essential to arrive at a satisfactory explanation of addiction. However, I am critical of his suggested relational ontology. Hill has done valuable work in pointing out natural scientific and abstractionist ontological foundations as the underlying paradigm of addiction studies, yet I do not believe that his proposed "relational ontology" provides an adequate solution to the problems of conceptual chaos and ineffectual treatment.

This book presents another option, which differs from Hill's (2010) relational ontology. Instead of proposing that the "conceptual confusion surrounding addiction is more apparent than real," and that there is "a shared unity at the ontological level" (p. 5), I propose that what creates the so-called "conceptual confusion" in addiction sciences is real from an epistemological perspective, and is a result of ontological reductionism. Furthermore, I do not entirely agree that most conceptions of addiction share a similar ontological basis (as suggested by Hill), and would prefer to state that each conception enacts a certain ontological reality and implies

---

[5] Boss (1983), in his book *The Existential Foundations of Medicine and Psychology*, provided a robust similar critique.

its own unique triadic relationship between ontology, epistemology, and methodology.

Hill (2010) identified the need for an alternative ontological viewpoint that "could offer a fresh approach to addiction and conceivably lead to greater treatment effectiveness" (p. 5). However, this seems viable only when placed in the above-mentioned triadic relationship. Moreover, it is also not clear how his alternative ontological viewpoint can provide conceptual integration.

In the next chapter I will argue that the solution is not to be found merely in a relational ontology, but rather in a pluralistic ontological and epistemological foundation. I propose that the application of integral theory as an epistemological and ontological (and methodological) foundation could provide an integrative conceptual framework, which could help address the problems of conceptual chaos and ineffectual treatment.

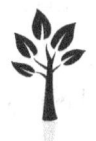

CHAPTER 3

Architectonic of an Integral Metatheory for Addiction

A new vision and understanding of something demands a new way of talking about it, for the old terminology gets in the way of this effort. Stubbornly entrenched behind the words coined by a particular conceptual orientation are its secret prejudices. Any attempt to open out an adequately human vista onto the phenomena of undisturbed existence must include a critique of the most important idea of traditional biology, physiology, and psychology.
—MEDARD BOSS (1983, P. 125)

INTRODUCTION

In the previous chapter, it was pointed out that the current state of addictionology presents a two-fold problem (Hill, 2010). Firstly, the cornucopia of theories and treatment methodologies appears to have resulted in confusion rather than cohesion and integration. Secondly, despite the wealth and variety of theoretical and treatment approaches to addiction, both researchers and clinicians recognize the failure of current interventions to produce significant effects at a population level; and it is clear that a paradigm shift is desperately needed in the field of addiction studies.

This paradigm shift would include alternative perspectives for studying human behavior (Reber & Osbeck, 2005; Richardson, 2005; Slife, 2005) like addiction (Du Plessis, 2013; Jay & Jay, 2000; Prentiss, 2005; Shaffer, 1995, 2007; White, 1998).

This book represents the beginning of one such an attempt at an alternative perspective of addiction, which may provide adequate conceptual integration, and that accounts for and integrates the multitude of etiological models, while not falling prey to the same disadvantages of the BPS model. In this chapter I will show how integral theory could possibly provide the conceptual architectonic for an integrative metatheory of addiction.

INTEGRAL THEORY

American philosopher Ken Wilber's (2000, 2006) integral theory is often referred to as the AQAL model, with AQAL representing all quadrants, all levels, all lines, all states and all types; these five elements signify some of the most basic repeating patterns of reality. Integral scholars believe that including all of these elements increases one's capacity to ensure that no major part of any solution is left out or neglected (Esbjörn-Hargens, 2009).

Integral theory is both complexifying in the sense that it includes and integrates more of reality and simplifying "in that it brings order to the cacophony of disparate dimensions of humans with great parsimony" (Marquis, 2009, p. 38). The strength of integral theory is its ability to integrate vast fields of knowledge. According to Marquis (2008), integral theory provides a "meta-theoretical framework that simultaneously honours the important contributions of a broad spectrum of epistemological outlooks while also acknowledging the parochial limitations and misconceptions of these perspectives" (p. 24). Wilber (2006) believes that integral theory is comprehensive rather than reductionist, and viewed it as "a comprehensive map of human potentials" (p. 1).

Integral theory has been applied in over 35 disciplines (Esbjörn-Hargens, 2006, 2009). The field of addiction studies and recovery is only one of these fields. Most of the articles published to date about the application of integral theory and substance abuse have focused on treatment design (Amodia, Cano, & Eliason, 2005; Du Plessis, 2010; 2012a; Dupuy & Gorman, 2010; Dupuy & Morelli, 2007; Nixon, 2012; Shealy, 2009) and only recently have articles exploring the application of integral theory in relation to etiological models of addiction been published (Du Plessis, 2012b, 2013, 2014a).

What makes integral theory particularly useful within the current context is its postmetaphysical stance and metatheoretical ability. Integral theory is "derived from the analysis of other theories, philosophies and cultural traditions of knowledge" (Edwards, 2008a, p. 65). It is important to point out that integral theory is not strictly a theory. In theory, data is the relevant set of empirical and conceptual experiences about which the theory makes some validity claim (Meehl, 1992). Integral theory is metatheoretical in that its elements are derived from the analysis of other theories. In other words, it "is not a theory because its subject matter is other theory and *not* the empirical world of immediate experience and the concepts and symbols that mediate those experiences" (Edwards, 2008a, p. 65). Edwards (2008a) further pointed out that integral theory, "has the capacity to adjudicate on how theories, and the core second-order conceptual elements that constitute them, relate to each other, how they appear in balanced or in distorted forms, and how they are combined to develop systems of knowledge, categories of social policy, and forms of practice that can either emancipate or enslave us and our communities" (p. 66).

Integral theory has been applied in integrally informed approaches to recovery (Amodia et al., 2005; Du Plessis, 2010, 2012a; 2012b; Dupuy &

Gorman, 2010; Dupuy & Morelli, 2007; Gorman, 2013; Nixon, 2012; Shealy, 2009) and tentative explorations of its relevance have been used to help understand the nature and etiology of addiction (Du Plessis, 2012b, 2013, 2014a). However, only preliminary academic research has been undertaken to explore the applicability of integral theory in the development of an integrative metatheory of addiction (Du Plessis, 2014b).

In previous research, the five elements of the AQAL model have been instrumental in developing integrally informed treatment protocols because of their consistency with empirical observation (Du Plessis, 2010; 2012a; Dupuy & Gorman, 2010). Although this application and analysis of the five elements of integral theory in relation to addiction and recovery is insightful and has assisted in treatment design, it is inadequate to provide a comprehensive schema of addiction or a comprehensive metatheory. Furthermore, many of the previous publications on integrally informed approaches to addiction fall prey to the same problems that Hill (2010) pointed out in his critique of the BPS model (Du Plessis, 2010, 2012a; Dupuy & Gorman, 2010; Dupuy & Morelli, 2007; Shealy, 2009).

However, the foundation for true conceptual integration could possibly be developed by means of a sophisticated application of integral theory's metaparadigmatic ability and its postmetaphysical stance. In the next sections we explore integral enactment theory and its application toward the development of an integrative metatheory of addiction.

Integral Enactment Theory

Integral scholar-practitioner, Sean Esbjörn-Hargens (2010) explained that at the core of integral enactment theory is the triadic notion of integral pluralism. He identified three pluralisms that are explicit within integral theory, namely, epistemological, methodological, and ontological. Integral pluralism points out that "epistemology is connected to ontology via methodologies. So, if we are going to have epistemological pluralism (the Who) and methodological pluralism (the How), then we ought logically (or integrally) to have ontological pluralism (the What)" (Esbjörn-Hargens & Zimmerman, 2009, p. 146).

Integral pluralism is composed of integral epistemological pluralism (IEP), integral methodological pluralism (IMP), and integral ontological pluralism (IOP) (Esbjörn-Hargens, 2010; Esbjörn-Hargens & Zimmerman, 2009). Before exploring the three facets of integral pluralism, the relevance of the concept of enactment, an essential feature of integral theory's postmetaphysical position, is discussed (Esbjörn-Hargens, 2010; Esbjörn-Hargens & Zimmerman, 2009; Wilber, 2003a, 2003b, 2006).

In this chapter I will discuss how integral enactment theory highlights the phenomenon of addiction as a multiple and dynamic object arising along a continuum of ontological complexity. Integral enactment theory adeptly points out how etiological models co-arise in relation to methodology (methodological pluralism) and enacts a particular reality of addiction (ontological pluralism), while being mediated by the worldview of the subject applying the method (epistemological pluralism).

Enactment

The idea of enactment is vital to understand why different theories of addiction do not have to contradict one another, as they are often interpreted, but can rather be understood as true but partial. Enactment is the bringing forth of certain aspects of reality (ontology) when using a certain lens (methodology) to view it (Esbjörn-Hargens, 2010).

In short, reality is not to be discovered as a pregiven truth, but rather reality is cocreated or coenacted by the various paradigms that are used to explore it (using the construct of a paradigm in the Kuhnian sense—which includes the social injunctions associated with a certain worldview). For example, when attempting to understand addiction using natural scientific research methods, a different ontological reality is enacted than when using a phenomenological approach. By avoiding what Wilber referred to as the "myth of the given," addiction is understood as a multiple object with no existing pregiven reality to be discovered (Wilber, 2003a, 2003b, 2006). Integral pluralism and its conception of enactment can be seen as a halfway position between subjective idealism or immaterialism and positivism or materialism.

> This is why I use the word sub-sist. There is a reality or a What that subsists and has intrinsic features but it doesn't ex-ist without a Who and a How. So that is where Integral Pluralism in general comes into being: it is bringing forth a reality but it is not creating the reality à la subjective idealism. (Wilber as cited in Esbjörn-Hargens, 2010, p. 169)

Different research methods in addictionology enact addiction in unique ways and consequently, bring forth different etiological models. Most of the etiological models, typically based on a positivist foundation, treat addiction as a single object "out there" to be discovered or uncovered and therefore, eventually run into trouble attempting to explain a feature of addiction outside of its enacted reality.

For example, physiological models and their accompanying research, namely, naturalistic scientific methodologies, enact the biological reality of addiction and are inherently incapable of showing any truth of addiction outside the realm of biology, that is, societal, existential, and so forth. In acknowledging the multiplicity of addiction's ontological existence, the incompatibility of the various etiological models disappears because we can see that each enacts a different reality of addiction—each brings forth valuable insights in its specific ontological domain. What one considers real depends in part on the means and apparatus one uses, so objects are, therefore, enacted (Murray, 2010).

In discussing the ontology of climate change, Esbjörn-Hargens (2010) raised some stimulating points. In explaining the inevitability of ontological pluralism of climate change, he pointed out a relationship between the various methods that are used to "see" or enact this complex phenomenon, namely, the relationship of (a) the common professions that encounter the phenomenon (the Who), (b) the associated methodology of each discipline (the How), and (c) the consequent view of climate change (the What). Exactly the same assertion can be made for the enactment of addiction models.

Applying the above-mentioned triadic relationship to the notion of addiction highlights some fascinating, but seldom acknowledged, issues. When the various professions explore etiological models and apply their respective methodologies, they may not refer to the same ontic phenomenon. It has often been acknowledged that various researchers and clinicians explore or treat different aspects of addiction, but often this is based on the assumption of a common ontic (and objective) reality of addiction and when "puzzled" together forms a comprehensive picture of addiction. This is the underlying ontological and epistemological assumption of the BPS model and other compound models. Is the above-mentioned a correct ontological assumption (What) on which to build theories (Why)? Is the neurobiologist seeing the same addiction as the existential therapist? Is the psychoanalyst talking about the same addiction as the Twelve Step counselor? Is the biochemist measuring the same addiction as the social scientist? Yes and no. Yes, in the sense that that they all attempt to view the socially defined and agreed-upon phenomena called addiction; and no, in the sense that they are "bringing-forth-into-the-world" and enacting different realities, ranging in ontological complexity (first, second, and third orders of ontology)—which can overlap ontologically, but are not the same ontic phenomenon.

In short, there are essential structures of addiction that share the various enactments of it, but how it "exists-in-the-world" varies, depending on the unique permutation of its integral enactment triad of "Who–How–What."

"In fact, there is not a clear, single, independently existing object, nor are there multiple different objects. There is something in-between: a multiple object. . . . This multiple object [addiction] is actually a complex set of phenomena that cannot easily be reduced to a single independent object" (Esbjörn-Hargens, 2010, p. 148).

The notion of enactment provides a lens of "ontological span" because it explains why different theories and their accompanying methodologies enact different aspects of an ontic phenomenon.

Integral Methodological Pluralism

Integral methodological pluralism (IMP) is derived from the eight zone extensions of the original AQAL model (Wilber, 2003a, 2003b, 2006). These eight primordial perspectives (8PP) are derived from an inside view (i.e., a first-person perspective) and an outside view (i.e., a third-person perspective) of the quadrants.

Each of the 8PP is only accessible through a particular method of inquiry or methodological family, and represents at least one of the eight most important methods for accessing reproducible knowledge (Esbjörn-Hargens, 2006, 2010). Furthermore, each of these methodologies discloses an aspect of reality unique to its particular injunction that other methods cannot. As such, IMP represents one of the most pragmatic and all-encompassing theoretical formulations of any integral or metatheoretical approach to accessing reproducible knowledge (Esbjörn-Hargens, 2006, 2010).

Wilber (2003b) believes that "any sort of Integral Methodological Pluralism allows the creation of a multi-purpose toolkit for approaching today's complex problems—individually, socially, and globally—with more comprehensive solutions that have a chance of actually making a difference" (p. 14).

IMP has two essential features: paradigmatic and metaparadigmatic. The paradigmatic aspect refers to the recognition, compilation, and implementation of all the existing methodologies in a comprehensive and inclusive manner. The metaparadigmatic aspect refers to its capacity to weave together and relate paradigms to each other from a metaperspective (Wilber, 2003b, 2006). Wilber (2003b) described the metaparadigmatic aspect of IMP as "a practice that can enact, bring forth, and illuminate the integral interrelationships between various holons originally thought discreet or non-existent" (p. 13). IMP can, therefore, be understood as the 8PP and its correlated methodologies with a metaframework, which provides metalinking between these disparate perspectives and paradigms (Martin, 2008).

The eight methodological families identified by Wilber (2003a, 2003b, 2006) are zone 1: phenomenology (the insides of individual interiors), zone 2: structuralism (the outsides of individual interiors), zone 3: hermeneutics (the insides of collective interiors), zone 4: cultural anthropology or ethnomethodology (the outsides of collective interiors), zone 5: autopoiesis theory (the insides of individual exteriors), zone 6: empiricism (the outsides of individual exteriors), zone 7: social autopoiesis theory (the insides of collective exteriors), and zone 8: systems theory (the outsides of collective exteriors). Wilber (2003a) used each of the names of these methodological families as an umbrella term, which includes many divergent and commonly used methodologies. These are depicted in Figure 1.

By using IMP, one "generates a meta-practice of honoring, including, and integrating the fundamental paradigms and methodologies of the major forms of human inquiry (traditional, modern, and postmodern)" (Wilber, 2003b, p. 16). By applying integral theory in the context of addiction models, one may be provided with a "meta-theoretical framework that simultaneously honours the important contributions of a broad spectrum of epistemological outlooks while also acknowledging the parochial limitations and misconceptions of these perspectives" (Marquis, 2008, p. 24).

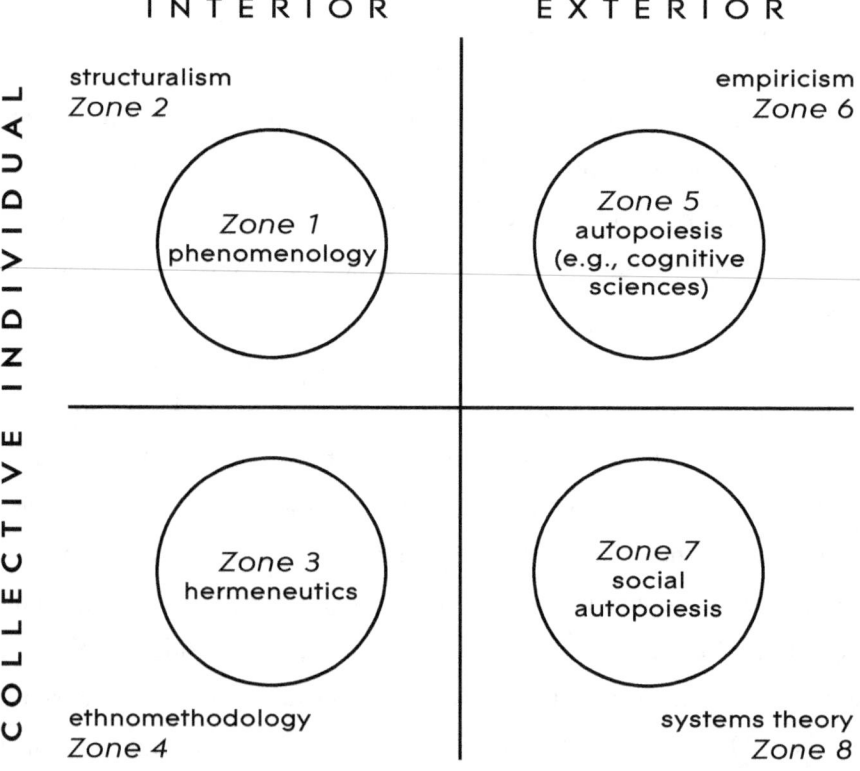

Figure 1: Eight methodological families of IMP. From "An Integral Ontology of Addiction: A multiple object existing as a continuum of ontological complexity," by Guy Du Plessis, 2014, *Journal of Integral Theory and Practice*, 9(1), p. 40. Reprinted with permission.

Integral taxonomy of etiological models of addiction

In Figure 2, an integrative taxonomy of etiological models of addiction (discussed in Chapter 1) is provided, using the eight zones and methodological families of IMP, into which etiological models can be grouped. By viewing addiction through the quadrants and its 8PP, one can see that all these perspectives with their respective methodological families need to be acknowledged, and as many as possible should be included in order to gain a truly comprehensive view. This avoids what Wilber (2006) referred to as "quadrant absolutism," where all realities of a phenomenon are reduced to the perspective of one quadrant, for example, reducing the multiple determinants of addictive behavior to merely impaired neurophysiology.

ZONE 1	ZONE 2	ZONE 3	ZONE 4
Phenomenology	**Structuralism**	**Hermeneutics**	**Ethnomethodology**
Conditioning/ Reinforcement Behavioral models Compulsion and Excessive Behavior models Spiritual/Altered State of Consciousness models Personality/Intrapsychic models Coping/Social learning models Biopsychosocial model	Transtheoretical model Personality/ Intrapsychic models	Coping/Social Learning models Biopsychosocial model	Social/Environment models Coping/Social Learning models Biopsychosocial model Spiritual/Altered State of Consciousness models

ZONE 5	ZONE 6	ZONE 7	ZONE 8
Autopoiesis theory	**Empiricism**	**Social autopoiesis theory**	**Systems theory**
Conditioning/ Reinforcement Behavioral models Coping/Social Learning models Biopsychosocial model	Genetic/Physiological models Conditioning/ Reinforcement Behavioral models Compulsion and Excessive Behaviour models Biopsychosocial model	Social/ Environment models	Social/Environment models Biopsychosocial model

Figure 2: Taxonomy of etiological models of addiction within the eight major methodological families of IMP. From "An Integral Ontology of Addiction: A multiple object existing as a continuum of ontological complexity," by Guy du Plessis, 2014, *Journal of Integral Theory and Practice*, 9(1), p. 43. Reprinted with permission.

By applying IMP to explanatory addiction models, it highlights how each of the single-factor models articulates addiction from a specific zone(s) because it applies a specific methodology, whereas the more integrative models view addiction across several of these zones. Each of the models indicated in Figure 2 brings valuable insight from a specific paradigmatic point of view and enacts certain features of addiction by virtue of applying particular methodologies. This pluralistic perceptive allows one to honor all the existing theories of addiction, and at the same time highlights their respective inadequacies.

From an IMP perspective, none of these models or perspectives has epistemological priority because they coarise and "tetra-mesh" simultaneously. Each of these explanatory models has advantages in describing certain features and etiological determinants of addiction, but also has limitations. Therefore, these models are valid from the perspectives they use to understand and study addiction, but are also always partial in their approach to the whole. From this perspective, a model is not correct or incorrect, but rather that it is more suited to explaining addiction from a certain perspective, and more limited from other perspectives. For instance, the genetic/physiological models are better at explaining the biological determinants and functions of addiction than the personality/intrapsychic models, whereas the personality/intrapsychic models are better at explaining the phenomenological determinants and experience of addicted individuals than the genetic/physiological models. Yet, both illuminate important and interlinked aspects of the same phenomenon.

Through the application of IMP, one can begin to develop a conceptual framework integration in which (a) all the evidence-based models are accounted for, (b) an explanation is given regarding which aspect of addiction they enact, and (c) metaparadigmatic integration of these diverse perspectives and their paradigmatic injunctions is provided.

It must be noted that IMP has to be placed within the larger context of integral pluralism. If this is not done, multiple perspectives (epistemological pluralism) are overemphasized (a mistake I made in previous research; see Du Plessis, 2012b) without recognizing that there are actually multiple objects (ontological pluralism) correlated with those perspectives and their respective methodologies (Du Plessis, 2013, 2014b; Esbjörn-Hargens, 2010).

Integral Epistemological Pluralism

Integral epistemological pluralism (IEP) refers to the multiplicity of perspectives or worldviews of how we can know a phenomenon. Each of the methodologies of IMP has a correlated epistemology. In other words, each method of studying addiction has its own belief regarding how we can know addiction. As already mentioned, IMP has to be placed within the larger context of integral pluralism.

> All too often we talk as if the multiple perspectives (e.g. worldviews represented by the altitudes) are all looking at the same object: epistemological pluralism . . . . If they all use the same method, then they might indeed enact a single object, but if they use very different methods, then the probability increases that they will enact a multiple object. (Esbjörn-Hargens, 2010, p. 155)

In short, not placing epistemological and methodological pluralism within the larger framework of integral pluralism tends to reinforce the myth of the given by implying a single "pre-given independent object" (Esbjörn-Hargens, 2010). Wilber (as cited in Esbjörn-Hargens, 2010) warned against the myth of the given by saying:

> There is no given world, not only because intersubjectivity is a constitutive part of objective and subjective realities, but also because even specifying intersubjectivity is not nearly enough to get over that myth in all its dimensions: you need to specify the Kosmic locations of both the perceiver and the perceived in order to be engaged in anything except metaphysics. (p. 150)

Murray (2012) pointed out that "Integral Pluralism says that what is perceived to exist depends on the methodology used to inquire and the developmentally-determined capacity of the observer/inquirer to perceive [epistemological pluralism]" (p. 35). Wilber's (2006) stages of development are an example of epistemological pluralism within integral enactment theory. From a moral developmental perspective, an easy way to understand stages is to describe their progression from egocentric (preconventional) through ethnocentric (conventional) to world-centric (postconventional). This is an example of how IEP accounts for a developmental understanding of addiction as well as recovery, and can account for the many empirical observations relating to addiction and the process of change described in developmental models such as the TTM (DiClemente, 2003).

In conclusion, the discussion suggests that when IEP is placed within the triadic relationship of integral pluralism, it reveals integral theory's capacity for conceptual integration and ontological span. In striving for conceptual integration, IEP highlights the underlying worldview or each model's injunction/methodology, which gives rise to a specific ontological understanding of addiction (ontological span).

Integral Ontological Pluralism

Philosophers have long pointed out that all concepts have ontological roots or make assumptions about the nature of reality (Bishop, 2007;

Polkinghorne, 2004; Slife, 2005). Addiction theories and definitions, like all scientific conceptions, and addiction treatments likewise begin with certain philosophical assumptions that determine the nature of the concept and how it may be applied (Bohman, 1993; Richardson, 2002; Slife, 2005). As indicated previously, in addictionology, these ontological assumptions often go unnoticed and consequently, unchallenged by researchers and clinicians when they begin to explore and treat the disorder (Hill, 2010; Shaffer, 1986).

Most addiction models, including the compound models, are not based on a pluralistic ontological foundation. This may be one of the pivotal reasons that conceptual integration has not yet been achieved in the addiction sciences. Ontological pluralism underscores that addiction is not a single pregiven entity, but rather a multiplicity of third-person realities. Moreover, the miscellany of the ontological realities of addiction has a special "enactive" relationship with etiological theories and their respective methodologies. Without acknowledging the ontological multiplicity of a complex phenomenon like addiction, conceptual integration cannot be achieved. Esbjörn-Hargens (2010) adds that "theory is not merely interpretive but constitutive: theoretical pluralism lends itself to ontological pluralism" (p.498). Esbjörn-Hargens (2010) described these relationships as "integral enactment." The relational scheme of integral enactment can be valuable in providing insight into the nature and genesis of etiological models of addiction.

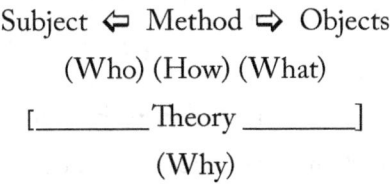

Figure 3: Integral enactment. From "An Ontology of Climate Change," by S. Esbjörn-Hargens, 2010, *Journal of Integral Theory and Practice*, 5(1), p. 157. Reprinted with permission.

In Figure 3, the relationships involved in integral enactment are shown. In short, etiological theories (Why) are part of an integral enactment of epistemology (Who), methodology (How), and ontology (What). Therefore, to understand why and how a model arrives at its ontological truth claims, all three of these elements need to be considered. Consideration of the elements will highlight what aspects of addiction the model can explain and what aspects it cannot.

The notion of addiction as a multiple ontological object may be one of the missing links in addiction science's goal to provide functional conceptual integration in the field. The perspective of integral ontological pluralism could help explain (and resolve) the difficulties encountered when attempting conceptual integration of explanatory models within a field as complex as addictions studies. It can account for conflicting empirical observations by incorporating an ontological pluralistic understanding of addiction. And it can highlight the ontological domain of research methodologies and their accompanied epistemologies. This can lead to various models not being understood as contradictory, but merely pointing to the different features of addiction on a continuum as a multiple object.

Addiction as a Third-Order Complexity

Ontological complexity can be a helpful notion in the quest for conceptual integration in the field of addiction studies. Esbjörn-Hargens (2010) described the three orders of complexity as follows:

> The first order is characterized by phenomena that we can more or less 'see' with our own senses. The second order is the result of using various extensions of our senses (instruments, computer programs, charts) to see the phenomena . . . . The third order cannot be seen with our senses nor indirectly by our instruments, but only by indications. (p. 159)

Addiction can thus be understood as a probability continuum of ontological complexity, co-arising and enacted through different methodologies and worldviews. At the highest level of abstraction (third-order) lies the notion of an individual's addiction-in-the-world, which is a staggeringly complex phenomenon beyond our senses or instruments. So addiction "is two steps removed from our direct experience (the first order) and our perception of it relies on many abstract indicators (the second order), which are epistemologically distant and ontologically complex" (Esbjörn-Hargens, 2010, p. 159).

When understanding addiction as a third-order ontology, we begin to understand why certain models of addiction, especially the single-factor models, give rise to such partial and reductionist explanations. They are good at explaining certain archaic features of addiction in the realm of its enacted first- or second-order ontology, but methodologically and epistemologically, they are incapable of enacting addiction on a third-order ontology. A perspective from a first- or second-order ontology cannot comprehensively articulate a complex phenomenon like addiction. Heather (as cited in West, 2005) pointed out certain features of the ontological complexity of addiction and the problem faced when etiological models do not include a perspective of ontological complexity:

> [A]ddiction . . . is best defined by repeated failures to refrain from drug use despite prior resolutions to do so. This definition is consistent with views of addiction that see decision-making, ambivalence and conflict as central features of the addict's behaviour and experience. On this basis, a three-level framework of required explanation is (needed) consisting of (1) the level of neuroadaptation [1st order ontology], (2) the level of desire for

drugs [2nd order ontology] and (3) the level of 'akrasia' or failures of resolve [3rd order ontology] . . . explanatory concepts used at the 'lower' levels in this framework can never be held to be sufficient as explanations at higher levels, i.e. the postulation of additional determinants is always required at Levels 2 and 3. In particular, it is a failure to address problems at the highest level in the framework that marks the inadequacy of most existing theories of addiction. (p. 2)

Most of the models discussed have as their foundation a natural scientific worldview and positivistic methodology that are typically adequate for exploring phenomena existing on the first- and second-order of ontological complexity. However, such models are hopelessly inadequate in explaining complex phenomena such as addiction (or any human behavior), which exist on the third order of ontological complexity. For example, reward deficiency syndrome (Blum, 1995) can only be understood as one of many possible physiological risks that interact with other aspects of being human, without having to reduce human behavior and motivation to neurotransmitter levels and brain metabolism. Simply put, even though an addict may have irregular brain metabolism and physiology, at the molecular realm of brain physiology, concepts such as addiction are meaningless.

In conclusion, the phenomenon of addiction is a third-order ontology, which can only be coenacted (brought-forth-in-the-world) when juxtaposed with associated methodological variety and epistemological depth (Esbjörn-Hargens, 2010). The notion of epistemological distance highlights that some facts of addiction speak louder than others and some elements of addiction are only enacted within certain worldviews. Methodological variety refers to the fact that:

> The more epistemological distance and ontological complexity increase, the more methodological variety will increase. Thus, the more multiple an object becomes (the What), the more methods and disciplines you will need to study and make sense of it (the How), and the more perspectives there will be on what is or is not the nature of that object (the Who). (Esbjörn-Hargens, 2010, p. 162)

IOP provides an ontological span and a pluralistic element, by clarifying the multiple object nature of addiction, whereas ontological complexity provides ontological depth by pointing out the various degrees of complexity each of these multiple objects can inhabit.

The value of an integral pluralism framework is that it provides a more accurate concept of how addiction is enacted—this right view lends itself to right action. The integral pluralism framework allows us to be more efficient in dealing with the various realities of addiction. This is because the integral enactment theory provides a more precise view of how addiction comes into being. "It will take many years to flesh out the details of this approach, but integral theory already offers us a substantial platform from which to begin enacting Integral Pluralism and developing an Integral Enactment Theory" (Esbjörn-Hargens, 2010, p. 165).

LENS-FIELD

To do justice to the total nature of man's being-in-the-world, I believe the metaphor of a lens often used in integral theory is too restrictive and unidirectional to symbolize the interdependent and coenactive nature of the epistemological/ontological/methodological pluralism it articulates. I prefer to use the metaphor of a "lens-field" epistemology when referring to ontic (in particular, human-being-in-the-world) phenomena, informed from the notion of field as described by philosopher-statesman Jan Smuts. Presaging integral theory's postmetaphysics,[6] Smuts (1926) conceptualized his notion of "fields" in his remarkable proto-integral book, *Holism and Evolution:*

> We have to return to the fluidity and plasticity of nature and experience in order to find the concepts of reality. When we do this we find that round every luminous point in experience there is a gradual shading off into haziness and obscurity. A "concept" is not merely its clear luminous centre, but embraces a surrounding sphere of meaning or influence of smaller or larger dimensions, in which the luminosity tails off and grows fainter until it disappears. Similarly a "thing" is not merely that which presents itself as such in clearest definite outline, but this central area is surrounded by a zone of intuitions and influences which shades off into the region of the indefinite. The hard abrupt contours of our ordinary conceptional system do not apply to reality and make reality inexplicable, not only in the case of causation, but in all cases of relations between things, qualities, and ideas. Conceive of a cause as a centre with a zone of activity or influence surrounding it and shading gradually off into indefiniteness . . . One of the most salutary reforms in

---

6   Integral theory as developed by Ken Wilber (1995, 2000) and other integral scholars acknowledge many antecedent foundational influences, and proto-integral thinkers. Curiously, South African philosopher and Commonwealth statesman, General Jan Smuts's (1926) theory of Holism is seldom acknowledged, although it has significantly contributed, albeit often implicitly, to the development of integral theory (Du Plessis, 2010; Edwards, 2003; Du Plessis & Weathers, 2015). Furthermore, Smuts's theory of holism also had a significant influence on scholars that integral thinkers point out as direct philosophical influences; though Smuts has been insufficiently acknowledged by contemporary integral scholars as an integral thinker in his own merit. It must be noted that Wilber (personal communication, July 21, 2009) does acknowledge Smuts's book *Holism and Evolution* as having a significant influence on his early thinking, but has not indicated this sentiment in his writings. I have previously (Du Plessis & Weathers, 2015) argued that Smuts should be counted among one of the great pioneering integral thinkers of the 20th Century.

thought which could be effected would be for people to accustom themselves to the ideal of fields, and to look upon every concrete thing or person or even abstract idea as merely a centre, surrounded by zones or aurae or spheres of the same nature as the centre, only more attenuated and shading off into indefiniteness. (pp. 17–19)

By using a lens-field epistemological metaphor and its relation to ontology, it highlights certain issues. Firstly, a lens-field enacts a specific ontological domain (or "luminous point") of a phenomenon, depending on its method of enquiry. Secondly, the enacted ontological domain (always a partial abstraction of its complete ontic boundaries) is seen rather as a field with a center of gravity (luminous point) enacted by a specific epistemology and methodology. Each enacted ontology will contain the fields of all other possible enacted ontologies of the full possible ontological nature of the phenomenon.

In the discussion about IMP, it was highlighted that different epistemological lenses with their accompanying methodologies enact different ontological realities of addiction. It was further pointed out that, according to the principles of integral enactment, none of these lenses has epistemological priority. However, without giving any lens-field epistemological priority as such, addiction (in the context of an individual) as an ontological reality has a certain center of gravity (luminous point) that is more clearly articulated by certain lens-fields than by others.

CRITIQUE OF INTEGRAL THEORY

A discussion of integral theory would not be complete without pointing out some thoughtful critiques. What follows is a succinct discussion, as it is beyond the scope of this book to provide an in-depth critique.

One critique that has been leveled against the integral model (as with other metatheories) is that there are few assessment measures in place for metatheory building. Science and the scientific method are chiefly linked with the empirical testing of theories rather than with their initial construction. Comparatively little programmatic research goes into theory building. Edwards (2013) expressed the opinion that while there has been much progress in metadata analysis, the other metalevel branches of study, the move toward a system of metastudies is only at a nascent stage of development.

What Edwards (2013) indicated is that since the integral model is essentially a metatheory, there are few measures in place to assess if integral theory is effective in building overarching metatheories or even to assess if integral theory itself is constructed successfully. Therefore, a critique can certainly be made that there is little research to test the validity of integral theory's metatheory building capacity as well as the soundness of its own metatheoretical foundation.

The neglect of method

Edwards (2013) expressed the view that "the neglect of method" is the most glaring problem that metatheoretical research faces. Ritzer (1991) and Skinner (1985), among others, have pointed out that metatheorising is a common preliminary research activity, yet has not been formalized. When researchers conduct a literature review they often engage in certain features of metatheorising.

According to Edwards (2013), "Metatheorising is still largely done surreptitiously or seen as the poor cousin to the real scientific task of theory testing. One reason for this devaluing of metatheoretical research has been the lack of formal research methods for carrying out meta-level research" (pp. 182–183). In addition, Edwards pointed out that for metatheoretical research to be accepted as good science it must assume systematic methods, appropriate research designs, and meticulous forms of analysis.

Idiosyncratic writing

Edwards (2008a, 2008b, 2013) has, in several articles, written about the weaknesses of the methodological approach used by Wilber (2006) as well as many other metatheorists because of the way in which they develop their overarching conceptual structures. He thus explained:

> Wilber and many other metatheorists rely on traditional scholarship methods of essentially reading a broad, but idiosyncratic, selection of writings and research and then making of it what they will according to their own assumptions and predilections. This traditional approach is not adequate if metatheoretical research is to be taken seriously as a form of social science research. (Edwards, 2013, p. 183)

Until the integral model develops a rigorous and methodological research activity it will, like many other metatheories, remain the idiosyncratic view of one visionary thinker and will have great difficulty in entering mainstream academia and being taken seriously by higher education institutions.

Epistemic fallacies

Murray (2010, 2011, 2012) made significant contributions in the field of integral theory by pointing out epistemic fallacies inherent in ontological schemes or models like integral theory. He astutely pointed out that integral theory needs to be packaged with an "indeterminacy analysis," which he correctly indicated is the job of the knowledge-building community and not of the originating theorist. The critique of integral theory can be understood as an indeterminacy analysis of integral theory's capacity to build an integrated metatheory of addiction, and what I call its "enactive capacity"; the latter is a model's inherent capacity to enact its observed ontological reality faithfully. Emphasis, here, is placed on degree, for as postmodern approaches have pointed out, it is unlikely that any ontological scheme can faithfully enact any ontological reality, without some conceptual distortion or coloring.

Murray (2012) highlighted epistemic drives within integral theory:

> Epistemic drives and various cognitive biases can lead to distorted or demi-real interpretations of reality. Concepts and ideas can be located along several spectra such as abstraction, 'ladder of inference', or emergent levels of reality. The further a concept is from concrete reality and observations (the further the epistemological distance), along any of these spectra, the more indeterminacy is involved and the greater the risk that there will be a mismatch in the structural properties of the idea vs. the structural properties of reality. (p. 36)

Previous sections have emphasized the value of ontological pluralism in relation to integral enactment theory. Murray (2012) made the critique that as with other aspects of integral theory, ontological pluralism lends itself to a positivist approach. Murray expressed the opinion that theories like Wilber's as well as the theories of other thinkers such as Bhaskar, Habermas, and Lakoff,

> were born in response to deconstructivist and poststructuralist approaches that, after rightly noting how knowledge is constructed and beliefs are strongly influenced by historical and sociocultural contingencies, went too far toward relativism and nihilism, completely dismissing the possibility of objective claims about reality. (p. 37)

Murray (2012) believed that that they have overcompensated "in their attempts to counterbalance the postmodern trends" (p. 37) by moving too far from postmodern insights, and avoiding and acknowledging "a deep consideration of the fallibility of knowledge and the indeterminacy of core concepts" (p. 37). This particular critique, that integral theory has gone too far in countering postmodern theories, was suggested by the subtitle of Gary Hampson's (2007) paper: "The [only] Way Out [of postmodernism] Is Through [it]."

Murray (2012) indicated how integral theory could "take some of its own medicine" by saying that:

> Integral Pluralism uses the idea of Ontological Pluralism to describe the indeterminacy of some controversial objects, such as climate change. What I am suggesting here is that it is useful to apply the concepts of Ontological Pluralism and metaphorical pluralism to the core abstract categories that comprise the theory itself. (p. 37)

Murray (2012) said that although "Wilber does employ various epistemic forms (as implied in 'tetra-enact') to indicate that the concepts and models he uses do not have a simple categorical form" (p. 50), it must, however, be noted that "in the vast majority of his writing and dialogue, he uses the categories without such qualification" (p. 50) and "when he notes the non-simplicity of the constructs" (p. 50) it is "not the same as noting the indeterminacies and fallibilities of the constructs themselves" (p. 50). For instance, the concepts of "The True," "the Good," and "the Beautiful," used by Wilber, often appear to be "given a foundational ontological status. But the True, the Good, and the Beautiful are metaphorical pluralisms that turn out to be difficult to pin down, and their meanings are contentious among philosophers" (Murray, p. 51).

In summary, Murray (2012) is of the opnion that integral theory contains enormously valuable ideas worth propagating extensively, but "integral theory could be packaged with an 'indeterminacy analysis' and other self-critical and self-reflective ideas that would make it easier for intermediate and advanced learners and practitioners to avoid the pitfalls of simple categorizations" (p. 52). Murray's statement has relevance for the project outlined in this book, and indicates that an indeterminacy analysis of the integral model will surely help to "avoid the pitfalls of simple categorisations" (p. 52) in attempting to develop a robust and functional integrated metatheory of addiction.

CONCLUSION

In this chapter I outlined how integral theory, in particular integral enactment theory, could possibly provide the conceptual architectonic for an integrative metatheory of addiction, which may assist with conceptual integration in the field of addiction studies.

The critiques raised against integral theory in this chapter are clearly valid, but they are not substantial enough to invalidate the use of integral theory in the development of an integrative metatheory of addiction.

In the next chapter I will explore how the five elements of the AQAL model can inform addiction treatment.

CHAPTER 4

Integral Addiction Treatment

Since Copernicus, man seems to have got himself on an inclined plane—now he is slipping faster and faster away from the center into—what? into nothingness? into a 'penetrating sense of his nothingness?' . . . . all science, natural as well as unnatural—which is what I call the self-critique of knowledge—has at present the object of dissuading man from his former respect for himself, as if this had been but a piece of bizarre conceit.
—FRIEDRICH NIETZSCHE (1887/1969, PP. 155–156)

INTRODUCTION

The conceptual chaos in the field of addiction research has direct implications for therapists working with addicted populations. For addiction treatment providers and therapists, it has become exceedingly difficult to integrate this vast and conflicting field of knowledge into effective treatment and prevention protocols.

Furthermore, it has been suggested that the low success rate for addiction treatment is because substance abuse programs apply partial and outdated treatment models (Du Plessis, 2010, 2012a, 2013; Jung, 2001; McPeak et al., 1991).

In this chapter[7], I will explore how the five basic elements of integral theory (Wilber, 2000, 2006) or the AQAL model (AQAL representing all quadrants, all levels, all lines, all states and all types) can inform addiction treatment. I will outline how integral theory can lay the foundation for a comprehensive and inclusive meta-therapeutic framework, referred to as an *integral meta-therapy*.

INTEGRAL THEORY

The Quadrants

According to integral theory, reality has at least four irreducible perspectives, which must be consulted when attempting to fully understand any aspect of reality: the subjective, intersubjective, objective, and interobjective (Esbjörn-Hargens, 2009). These four universal perspectives are known as the quadrants. In previous articles, researchers have pointed out that any treatment program will be incomplete if it does not account for all four quadrants in its therapeutic understanding and design (Amodia et al., 2005; Du Plessis, 2010, 2012a, 2012b, 2013, 2014a; Dupuy & Gorman, 2010; Dupuy & Morelli, 2007; Gorman, 2013; Shealy, 2009). In the following section of the chapter I will explore addiction and its treatment from each of these four perspectives.

---

7 The content of this chapter is adapted from previous publications, reprinted with permission (see Du Plessis, 2010, 2012a, 2012b).

Chapter 4: Integral Addiction Treatment

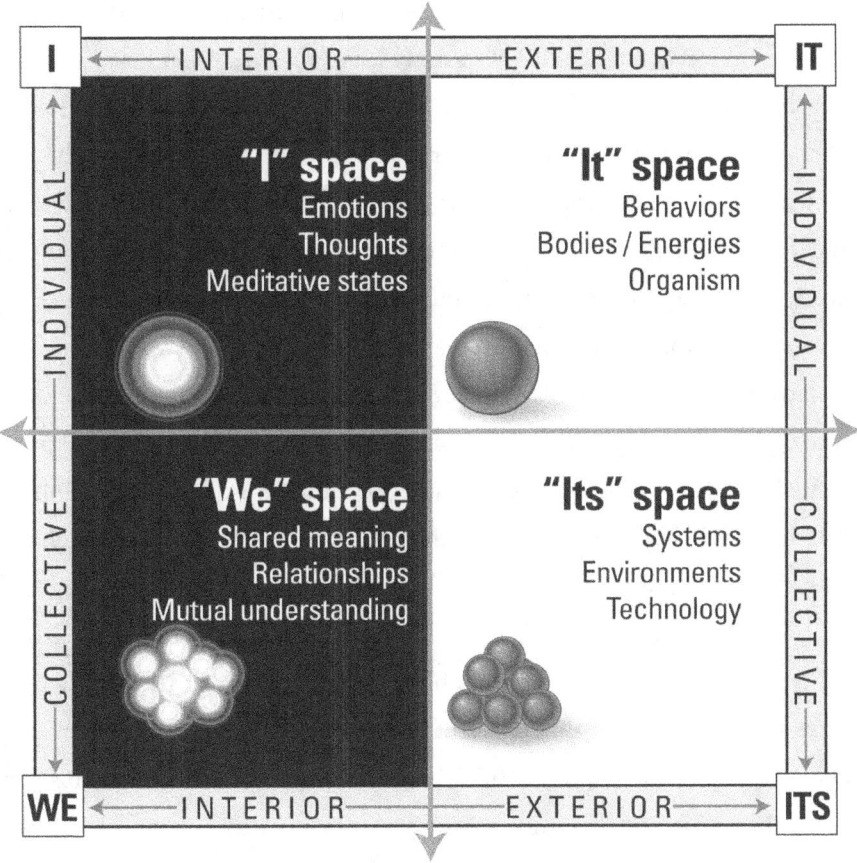

Figure 4: The quadrants. From "An Integral Guide to Recovery: Twelve Steps and Beyond". Guy du Plessis, 2015, Tuscon, AZ: Integral Publishers, p. 14. Reprinted with permission.

Upper-Right Quadrant

In attempting to understand addiction and recovery through exploring objective aspects of an individual—from the upper-right quadrant perspective—we notice all the positivistic and objective perspectives of individual structures, events, behaviors, and processes (Marquis, 2008).

From this perspective, addiction is viewed as dysfunctional brain physiology. Addiction affects the mesolimbic system of the brain, the area where our instinctual drives and our ability to experience emotions and pleasure reside. The medial forebrain bundle, popularly known as the "pleasure pathway" is in this area (Brick & Erickson, 1999). The pleasure pathway of the brain is "hijacked" by the chronic use of drugs or compulsive addictive behavior. As a result of the consequent neurochemical dysfunction, the individual perceives the drug as a life-supporting necessity, much like breathing or meeting the demands of thirst or hunger (Brick & Erickson, 1999).

As addiction affects both physical and neurological well-being, an effective recovery model needs to address these areas. Holford, Miller, and Braly (2008) emphasized the importance of diet and nutritional supplements in treating addictions and in the maintenance of recovery. Holford et al. believed that most addicts suffer from reward deficiency, which is a neurochemical imbalance in brain chemistry that translates into negative emotions such as anxiety, feelings of emptiness, and hypersensitivity. Many addicts have deficiencies in brain chemistry even prior to their addiction. There are many factors that can create a reward-deficient brain chemistry such as genetics, prenatal conditioning, malnutrition, stress, lack of sleep, physical or emotional trauma, and the long-term use of mood-altering substances. If not rectified, this brain chemistry deficiency will continue indefinitely through an addict's recovery period, resulting in recovering addicts being prone to relapse, even though they are abstinent and doing psycho-spiritual work. The symptoms of reward deficiency only abate when the neurochemical imbalance is corrected. Erickson (1989) suggested that for treatment to be effective, a combined physiological and psychological approach is required and without improving an addict's neurophysiology, treatment is often fruitless or incomplete.

It is indubitable that addiction has a significant biological component, but to reduce addiction to neurophysiology (for example the "brain disease" model) is a gross error. The reason this way of thinking is so readily accepted is that it is congruent with the prevailing scientific materialistic worldview that dominates most analyses of addiction and human behavior. Simply put, viewing addiction primarily as biology is making an error in assigning addiction an ontological status that is not befitting of its true complexity.

Upper-Left Quadrant

Exploring addiction and recovery from the Upper-Left Quadrant perspective includes the subjective dimensions of individual consciousness. Addiction wreaks havoc in the addict's inner phenomenal world and has disastrous consequences for the addict cognitively, existentially, and emotionally. The addict starts to lose control of his or her inner world as the "addict voice" becomes progressively louder. Addiction is progressive and will eventually negatively alter the interior phenomenal world of the addict. Nakken (1998) expressed the view that addiction develops from a definite, though often seemingly indistinct beginning, towards a specific end-point. The end-point of the addictive process is complete control of the self by the illness.

Addicts are known to have turbulent and overwhelming inner worlds. From a psychodynamic perspective, addiction is often referred to as an attempt at self-medicating the addict's painful and confused inner world (Khantzian, 1999). Owing to defects in ego and self-capacities, the substance of choice becomes the addict's main method of mood management, which temporarily restores inner equilibrium. Flores (1997) believes that addiction can be

> viewed as a misguided attempt at self-repair. Because of unmet developmental needs, certain individuals will be left with an injured, enfeebled, uncohesive, or fragmented self . . . alcohol, drugs, and other external sources of gratification (i.e., food, sex, work, etc.) take

on a regulating function while creating a false sense of autonomy, independence, and denial of need for others. (p. 233)

Therefore, an essential component of recovery is learning healthy ways to self-soothe and to cope with stress (Khantzian, 1999; Levin, 1995). If not addressed, these individuals will continue to seek dysfunctional ways to deal with their turbulent inner worlds, ineffective object-relations, and unresolved trauma (Flores, 1997).

A vital component of a comprehensive therapeutic protocol is some form of psychotherapeutic process that deals with unresolved trauma, family-of-origin issues, shadow work, and the building of emotional literacy. According to Ulman and Paul (2006), psychotherapy can serve as a transitional self-object, dispensing functions that serve as "psychopharmacotherapeutic" relief. In other words, a psychotherapist can replace the faulty self-object-like functioning of a client's drug of choice, and help the client to reexperience "archaic moods of narcissistic bliss" (Ulman & Paul, 2006) in a therapeutic, rather than an addictive fashion: "Such an altered state of consciousness may eventually supersede and supplant an addicted patient's dependence on an addictive state of mind" (p. 63).

In a letter addressed to Bill Wilson, the cofounder of AA, Carl Jung wrote: "You see, alcohol in Latin is *spiritus* and you use the same word for the highest religious experience as well as for the most depraving poison. The helpful formula therefore is: *spiritus contra spiritum*" (as cited in Kurtz & Ketcham, 2002, p. 118). Jung was pointing out to Wilson that at the heart of a cure for alcoholism there often is a spiritual transformation, because he also believed that the thirst for alcohol "was the equivalent, on a low level, of the spiritual thirst of our being for wholeness, expressed in medieval language: the union with God" (Jung, as cited in Kurtz & Ketcham, p. 113). Due to the influence of Carl Jung and others such as William James, AA and subsequent Twelve Step groups have seen the need for healthy spirituality as a central component of the recovery process (Kurtz & Ketcham, 2002).[8]

Rioux (1996) illustrated how certain spiritual healing techniques can play a role in a holistic addiction counseling approach as they focus on inner realities that produce harmony and self-wholeness. Winkelman (2001) further suggested that spiritual practices can also free addicts from ego-bound emotions and provide balance for conflicting internal energies. Spiritual practices can help addicts achieve a sense of wholeness to counter the sense of self-loss, which lies at the core of addictive dynamics. These practices enhance self-esteem by providing connectedness beyond the egoic self, with a "higher power of your understanding" as suggested in Twelve Step programs.

Addicts often relate that the initial pull toward drugs was the perceived meaningless of their own lives and the instant sense of meaning that drugs as well as drug culture provided. Jungian analyst Luigi Zoja is of the opinion that "one often turns to drugs because of the insignificance, senseless and flatness of one's present life, a dead and senseless thing fuelled by solely reflex action" (1989, p. 58). Viktor Frankl (1953), the founder of logotherapy, said a human being's most basic motivation is to find meaning in life. He believed other motivations are secondary to this primary motivation and lack of such purpose leads to a sense of frustration, emptiness, and in some cases, addiction.

---

8   The centrality of spirituality in current treatment programs can be problematic. Underlying these spiritually-orientated treatment approaches is a belief that a successful recovery program must contain a spiritual component and that spirituality is an innate feature of our being-in-the-world. I believe this view is misguided. I do not want to underplay the usefulness or even the necessity of spirituality in many people's lives, but I do not believe that spirituality is ontological in the sense that it is an essential need, but rather an essential need underlies it—the need for personal and global meaning. Spirituality or religion is often a vehicle for this need, but personal and global meaning can also be found within a secular worldview. For those with a secular worldview or for those not inclined toward spiritual/religious practice, any pursuit(s) that provides meaning is adequate to satisfy their existential need for meaning.

Lower-Left Quadrant

Understanding addiction and recovery from the Lower-Left Quadrant, the "we" space or perspective includes the intersubjective dimension of the collective (Marquis, 2008). Addiction progressively erodes relationships and is often caused by eroded relationships. Addiction may be viewed as an intimacy disorder as addicts often have an inability to form healthy intimate relationships (Carnes, 2008).

Eventually, many addicts undergo a cultural shift and enter the world of addiction with its own rules and cultural norms. Addicts find themselves in a new culture where their addictive behaviors are accepted and often encouraged. "The physiological, psychological, and spiritual transformations that accompany the person-drug relationship occur within and are shaped by the culture of addiction" (William White, 1996, p. xxiii).

William Burroughs (as cited in White, 1996) said the following about heroin addiction: "Junk is not just a habit. It is a way of life. When you give up junk, you give up a way of life" (p. 2). It is these cultural and relational aspects of addiction, this way of life, that many addicts find the hardest to give up. Any form of treatment that does not acknowledge and understand the principles behind the culture of addiction as well as the need for a healthy recovery culture is bound to be ineffective. "Addiction and recovery are more than something that happens inside someone. Each involves deep human needs in interaction with a social environment. For addicts, addiction provides a valued cocoon where these needs can be, and historically have been met" (White, 1996, p. xxvi).

Scholars who support the self-medication hypothesis believe that addicts often suffer from defects in their psychic structure as a result of poor relationships when they were young (Flores, 1997; Khantzian et al., 1990; Levin, 1995). This leaves them prone to seek external sources of gratification such as drugs, sex, food, and work in later life (Kohut, 1971, 1977). Khantzian (1999) asserted that "substance abusers are predisposed to become dependent on drugs because they suffer with psychiatric disturbances and painful affect states. Their distress and suffering is the consequence of defects in ego and self capacities which leave such behaviour" (p. 1).

For addicts to develop a healthy and stable sense of self, they need to be in a supportive and knowledgeable social environment. The addict's psychic troubles are born from poor relationships and can only be modified through new relationships (Khantzian, 1999 Kohut, 1977; Kurtz, 1982). Some object-relation theorists believe Twelve Step fellowships provide the ideal social environment for addicts to heal their psychic deficits (Flores, 1997).

Lower-Right Quadrant

Exploring addiction and recovery from the Lower-Right Quadrant includes the interobjective perspective of systems, addressing observable aspects of societies such as economic structures, civic resources, and geopolitical infrastructures (Marquis, 2008). Addiction affects this realm profoundly. Addicts often lose their jobs, get evicted, get into trouble with the law, and may be incarcerated. While there are many acultural addicts who manage to keep their jobs and have financial stability, for the majority of addicts this quadrant is severely compromised.

The culture of addiction has its own infrastructure—crack houses, bars, night clubs, casinos, strip clubs, and such. As addicts progressively migrate from one culture to the next, they start spending more time within the infrastructure of addiction culture. The more addicts frequent and live within the infrastructure of the culture of addiction, the more their behavior is normalized, which ultimately reinforces their denial of the problem. An essential component of treatment is addressing the damage done by addiction in this quadrant.

Lines of Development

According to integral theory, each aspect of the quadrants has distinct capacities that progress developmentally; these are known as lines of development (Esbjörn-Hargens, 2009). Wilber (2000) has theorized that each person has multiple lines of development, similar to Howard Gardner's (1993) conception of multiple intelligences. Each quadrant comprises many lines of development; for example, the Upper-Left Quadrant includes cognitive, emotional intelligence, spiritual, moral, interpersonal, and so forth. Although the concept of multiple lines of development is a nondominant notion in developmental psychology and empirical proof for separate lines of development is inconclusive, it nevertheless remains a useful clinical metaphor (Forman, 2010; Ingersoll & Zeitler, 2010).

A lines of development perspective highlights the fact that an individual's recovery process has distinct, yet interrelated, components that can be at different stages of development. Viewing the recovery process from a lines of development perspective provides insight for therapists and clients as to what aspects of the client's recovery program is doing well and what can be improved.

Stages of Development

An individual's lines of development can be understood to fluctuate through a sequence of developmental altitudes, known in integral theory as stages or levels of development (Wilber, 2006). An insight into addiction and recovery from a stage perspective is imperative for truly all-inclusive understanding and treatment (Du Plessis, 2010, 2012a; Dupuy & Gorman, 2010; Dupuy & Morelli, 2007).

A therapist could incorporate three types of developmental stage models into his or her therapeutic orientation. The first is the client's general stage of development (Cook-Greuter, 2004; Gruber & Voneche, 1977; Wilber, 2006). A client's overall development or center of gravity "is a key factor in treatment planning, profoundly influencing which categories of intervention are likely to be optimal, neutral, or contraindicated" (Marquis, 2009, p. 18). The second type is the client's stage of change as defined by the transtheoretical model of intentional behaviour change (DiClemente & Prochaska,

1998). Finally, the third type is the general attitude of a client to recovery based on clean time and stage of recovery using recovery-based developmental approaches (Bowden & Gravitz, 1998; Du Plessis, 2012b; Nakken, 1998; Whitfield, 1991). Depending on the client's stages of development, various recovery practices and therapies are suggested.

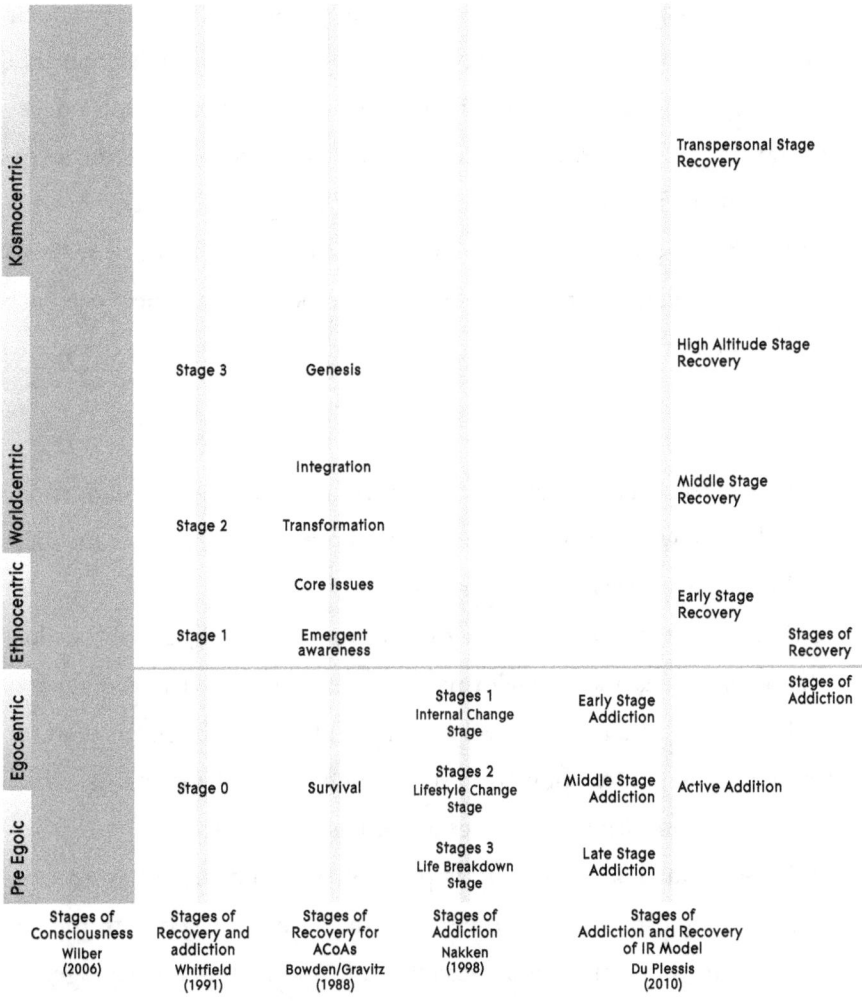

Figure 5: Developmental models of addiction and recovery. From "Integrated Recovery Therapy: Toward an integrally informed individual psychotherapy for addicted populations," by Guy du Plessis, 2012a, *Journal of Integral Theory and Practice*, 7(1), p. 130. Reprinted with permission.

In Figure 5, the developmental model used in integral theory, developmental models of addiction and recovery, as well as my own composite developmental model is depicted (Du Plessis, 2012b). Although the stages of addiction and recovery may be better understood as chronological stages or phases, there may be a correlation between the stage model as articulated in integral theory and the various stages (or phases) of recovery models. Simply put, earlier stages of recovery may correlate with early developmental stages and later stages of recovery may correlate with more complex developmental stages. The figure is a simplification of the developmental stages at which a client's "center of recovery gravity" can possibly rest. It must be noted that the figure is speculative regarding how the stages of recovery and addiction relate to other developmental models, and is best used as a clinical metaphor.

Recovery Stages

The stages of recovery indicated on the far right in Figure 5 are understood in the following way: Early stage recovery refers to the stage where the focus is on abstinence and relapse prevention.

Middle-stage recovery is where the focus is on working through various psychological issues and behavior patterns that often predate the onset of addiction. In this stage of recovery, many addicts also begin to work on codependency issues, relationship issues, and behavioral addictions, which tend to surface once their substance abuse has been addressed.

High-altitude stage recovery is perhaps best understood as an existentially-oriented stage, where the recovering addict is faced with life and social concerns that transcend issues related to addiction. At this stage, the distinction between addict and nonaddict begins to fall away. A recovery lifestyle will share similarities with the lifestyle of any individual at a similar stage of development. This is also the stage where the concept of fellowship begins to have a much more inclusive scope than merely Twelve Step fellowships.

The transpersonal stage of recovery can be understood as a stage that requires a special type of practice and orientation to attain. This developmental stage of recovery is normally reserved for those that have engaged in a significant amount of contemplative practices.

Clinical social worker and researcher Gary Nixon (2012) has written extensively about stages of recovery and suggested that the recovery process can be understood in three stages, similar to my addiction/recovery stage model discussed above. In Stage 1, the focus is on abstinence from alcohol and drugs. This stage correlates with what I refer to as early stage recovery. In Stage 2, similar to my middle stage recovery,

> The behavioral abstinence of stage one recovery can be enhanced by working through a range of prepersonal and personal emotional issues of stage two recovery, such as dissolving the false core driver and reestablishing basic trust, reintegrating the shadow, dismantling the internal critic, burning though social anxiety and co-dependency patterns, dismantling the crystallized ego, and embracing existential issues of meaning and authenticity. (Nixon, 2012, p. 245)

In Stage 3, which I call the transpersonal stage of recovery (see Figure 5), Nixon (2012) applied Wilber's ego-transcendence transpersonal levels, and points out that:

> Clients learn to let go of their separate self egos in each moment to embrace nondual living and become fully integrated beings. The long journey of transformation turns from the initial descent of addiction to a wondrous beingness of moment to

moment existence for the person who has now fully embraced stage three recovery. (p. 245)

In my addiction/recovery developmental model, as pointed out previously, I included a level of development referred to as high-altitude stage recovery between Nixon's Stage 2 and Stage 3 of recovery.

What Nixon (2012) referred to as Stage 1 and Stage 2 recovery, and what I refer to as early- and middle-stage recovery, is fairly well-articulated in recovery literature and there is significant guidance for those at these stages. On the other hand, there is very little guidance for those who are at a high-altitude stage or for those at a Stage 3/transpersonal stage of recovery. At a high-altitude stage and at a Stage 3/transpersonal stage of recovery, it now becomes the recovering addict's responsibility to seek guidance beyond the confines of traditional recovery literature and fellowship. There are many communities and teachers that can assist in these stages of development. The integral community is one such example. It is encouraging to see, for many recovering addicts entering these stages of development, that there is recovery literature emerging that is beginning to address these higher stages of recovery.[9]

A drawback of not viewing the recovery journey from a developmental perspective is thinking that recovery is about reaching the "recovery nirvana," often referred to as "serenity" in Twelve Step fellowships. This is not to say that recovering addicts do not become more serene, but rather that there is no final place of "ultimate serenity." Developmental theories enlighten us to the fact that each new stage brings forth its own rewards, challenges, and possible pathologies. Moreover, each new stage requires more sophisticated

---

9 See Gary Nixon's book, *The Sun Rises in the Evening*, John Dupuy's book, *Integral Recovery*, Robert Weathers' soon-to-be published book, *Plural Recovery: Integrally Informed Therapy and Relapse Prevention for Couples*, and my book, *An Integral Guide to Recovery: Twelve Steps and Beyond*.

recovery technology to be able to navigate the new stage adequately. If we look at this phenomenon from a developmental perspective, it is obvious why: The recovery practices, which worked at a previous stage will not be effective at a new stage. They may still have many benefits, but they need to be augmented to be effective at the higher recovery stage.

States of Consciousness

"In addition to levels and lines there are also various kind of states associated with each quadrant. States are temporary occurrences of aspects of reality" (Esbjörn-Hargens, 2009, p. 13). Understanding addiction and recovery from a state perspective may be one of the missing links in contemporary addiction treatment programs' attempts to create sustainable treatment protocols. Addicts are obviously experts on states. Using substances or engaging in any mind-altering behavior is an attempt to create an altered state of consciousness (ASC), and the specific psychoactive effect of various drugs and mind-altering behavior creates various types of ASCs (Milkman & Sunderworth, 2010). It follows that viewing addiction in terms of an ASC perspective is crucial for a complete understanding of the nature of addiction (Winkelman, 2001).

Some researchers have argued that the majority of addiction treatment programs fail to integrate a huge body of literature that highlights the therapeutic benefits for addicts in experiencing ASCs. They propose that a principal reason for the high relapse rate in treatment programs is the failure of those programs to address the basic need to achieve ASCs (McPeak et al., 1991). Some scholars believe that humans have an innate drive to seek ASCs (e.g., McPeak et al., 1991; Weil, 1972; Winkelman, 2001; K. Wilber, personal communication, January 13, 2011). They believe that addicts follow a normal human motive to achieve ASCs, but they use maladaptive methods because they are not provided with the opportunity to learn "constructive alternative methods for experiencing non-ordinary consciousness" (McPeak, as cited in Winkelman, 2001, p. 340). From this viewpoint, substance use is not understood as a pathology, but rather as a yearning to have a basic human need met.

AA acknowledges the importance of an alteration of consciousness for recovery to be effective: It calls for "a new state of consciousness and being" (Alcoholics Anonymous, 1987, p. 106) designed to replace the self-destructive pursuit of alcohol-induced states with a healthier life-enhancing approach. AA advocates meditation, a change in consciousness, and spiritual awakening as fundamental to achieve and maintain sobriety.

Blum (1995) expressed the opinion that addicts often have a neurologically based inability to experience pleasant feelings within simple life experiences and suggested that a neurological-normalizing shift may happen as a result of neurotherapy, which rectifies the endless quest for neurotransmitter balance; the latter is explained in his reward deficiency syndrome model.

Every human being engages in various activities to feel good. Feeling good and avoiding unnecessary pain are universal needs. To feel good, we seek out activities that alter our brain chemistry. Addiction can be understood as this normal need gone awry. Milkman and Sunderworth (2010) stated, "In light of the seemingly universal need to seek out altered states, it behooves researchers, educators, parents, politicians, public health administrators, and treatment practitioners to promote healthy means to alter brain chemistry" (p. 6). Addicts have found a dysfunctional way to meet this innate need through substances or certain behaviors to which they become addicted. Addicts normally have three dominant ways of seeking comfort and altering their consciousness:

> We repeatedly pursue three avenues of experience as antidotes for psychic pain. These preferred styles of coping—satiation, arousal, and

fantasy—may have their origins in the first years of life. Childhood experiences combined with genetic predisposition are the foundations of adult compulsion. The drug group of choice —depressants, stimulants, or hallucinogens—is the one that best fits the individual's characteristic way of coping with stress or feelings of unworthiness. People do not become addicted to drugs or mood-altering activities as such, but rather to the satiation, arousal, or fantasy experiences that can be achieved through them. (Milkman & Sunderworth, p. 19)

The quotation above clearly points to the need for addicts in recovery to find healthy behaviors and activities to manifest their preferred coping style since this preferred coping style (satiation, arousal, or fantasy) often correlates with their drug of choice (Du Plessis, 2012a).

Types

"The notion of types in the Integral model describes the diverse styles that a person (UL or LL) may use to translate or construct reality within a given stage of development" (Forman, 2010, p. 231). Esbjörn-Hargens (2009) added, "Types are the variety of consistent styles that arise in various domains and occur irrespective of developmental levels. As with the other elements, types have expression in all four quadrants" (p. 15). We can, therefore, have various classifications of different types in the context of addiction and recovery in each of the four quadrants: types of substance use disorders such as alcohol use disorder, stimulant use disorder, opioid use disorder; types of cultural enmeshment, for example acultural, bicultural, and culturally enmeshed; types of dual-diagnosis; types of kinship in subcultures; DSM-5 disorder types; and many more.

The usefulness of viewing addiction and recovery from a typology perspective is illustrated in the following two examples. First, in the discussion of states, we see that among addicts there are typically three different types of coping styles, namely, satiation, arousal, or fantasy that correlate with their drug of choice: depressants, stimulants, or hallucinogens.

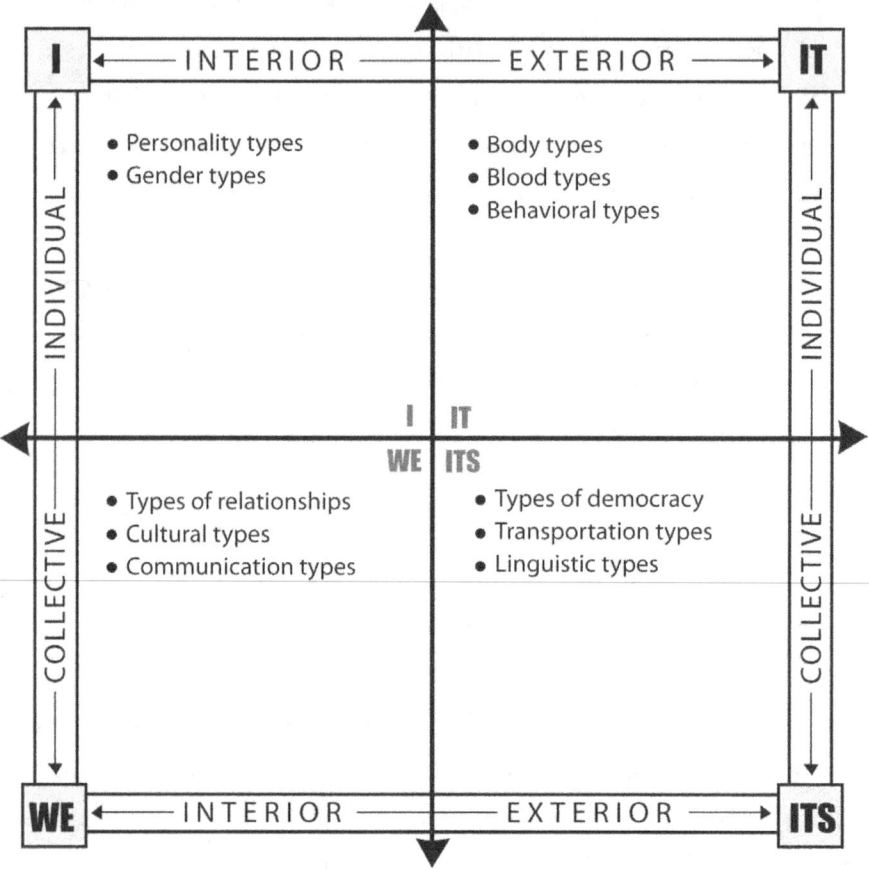

Figure 6: Typologies in the quadrants

Milkman and Sunderworth (2010) stated, "After studying the life histories of drug abusers, we have seen that drugs of choice are harmonious with an individual's usual means of coping with stress" (p. 19). Applying this simple typology to a client's drug of choice informs the therapist regarding a number of important factors. It enables the therapist to identify the client's primary mode of stress reduction by correlating it to his or her drug of choice.

When in recovery, the client will continue to use a preferred coping style and will be attracted to activities that produce a similar effect to his or her drug of choice. For example, an amphetamine user will likely be attracted to high-risk, physically demanding activities that are stimulating.

Another useful typology is the bioself-psychological typology of addiction of Ulman and Paul (2006), which is a synthesis of the self-psychological and biological-psychiatric versions of bipolarity. Kohut (as cited in Ulman and Paul, 2006) whose concept of the bipolar self, represents the foundation for Ulman and Paul's model stated:

> The self should be conceptualized as a lifelong arc linking two polar sets of experiences: on one side, a pole of ambitions related to the original grandiosity as it was affirmed by the mirroring self-object, more often the mother; on the other side, a pole of idealizations, the person's realized goals, which, particularly in the boy though not always, are laid down from the original relationship to the self-object that is represented by the father and his greatness. (p. 30)

In the bioself-psychological typology, addiction is understood as a psychological end result of developmental arrest in the bipolarity of the formation of the self. Biological psychiatrists, in their conception of bipolar spectrum disorder, devote considerable attention to depression and mania as they manifest in this disorder. These mood disorders correlate with disorders of the bipolar self as understood by Kohut (in Ulman & Paul, 2006):

> In general, a disturbance in the pole of grandiosity may find expression in either an empty, depleted depression or, in contrast, in over-expansive and over-exuberant mania or hypomania; whereas

a disturbance in the pole of omnipotence may appear in either depressive disillusionment and disappointment in the idealized or, in contrast, in manic (or hypomanic) delusions of superhuman physical and/or mental powers. We maintain that an individual maybe subject to specific outcomes resulting from a disturbance in either or both of these poles of the self. (pp. 395–396)

Owing to the specific accompanying mood disorder of each of the possible disturbances of the poles of the self, individuals will be attracted to certain psychoactive substances, which can be understood as an unconscious attempt at rectifying a specific deficit in self and coping style (Ulman & Paul, 2006).

There are many personality types that can be applied in the context of addiction and recovery. One example is that of feminine and masculine types. "When we speak of 'masculine' and 'feminine' we are not necessarily speaking of biological 'male' or 'female'. Rather we are referring to a spectrum of attitudes, behaviors, cognitive styles, and emotional energies" (Dupuy & Morelli, 2007, p. 37). The psychoactive properties of drugs and even aspects of process addictions can have a masculine or feminine "voice." "Downers" such as tranquilizers, barbiturates, and heroin can be understood as having a feminine voice, and moreover, addictions such as codependency, love addiction, certain aspects of sex addiction, and certain aspects of gambling (particularly slot machines) have a similar voice. On the other hand, "uppers" such as cocaine, methamphetamine, and process addictions such as certain high-risk aspects of sex addiction and gambling (especially gamblers who play tables) have a more masculine voice (Du Plessis, 2010, 2012a).

Using the masculine and feminine typology, we can see how the psychopharmacological properties of certain classes of psychoactive substances correlate with masculine and feminine typologies (i.e., depressants/feminine and stimulants/masculine), and how these poles of the self can also be classified within a masculine and feminine typology (pole of grandiosity/feminine and pole of idealizations/masculine). We can, therefore, see how certain "masculine" or "feminine" drugs act as a structural prosthesis in an attempt to rectify dysfunctional masculine or feminine poles of the self and coping styles (Du Plessis, 2010). Furthermore, I have observed that there seems to be a correlation between the quality of an addict's early relationships with their caregivers and their drug(s) of choice (Kernberg, 1975; Kohut, 1977).

Understanding the voice of the addiction can help in choosing an appropriate therapeutic treatment plan. Furthermore, some addictions only function in the dialectic between the masculine and feminine voices, that is, the alcoholic and the codependent enabler, the dance of the love addict and the love avoidant. It is important for the treatment professional to know which voice has become pathological and to bring that voice back into healthy balance.

TOWARD AN INTEGRAL META-THERAPY

Applying an integral foundation to therapy is not the same as methodology. An integral framework merely provides the conceptual scaffolding for a therapist, but does not indicate what methodology to use. It merely illuminates the territory. It would be inaccurate to think that an integral framework is going to improve poor therapeutic skills or make inadequate methodologies effective. Therefore, applying integral theory to therapy is best understood as a meta-therapy, in the sense that it provides a multiperspectival and metatheoretical perspective of the therapeutic process when guiding addicted clients in their recovery process.

As shown in this chapter, an integral meta-therapy will apply the five conceptual lenses of integral theory in the therapeutic process. An integral meta-therapy for addicted populations will have two main features, paradigmatic and metaparadigmatic. The paradigmatic aspect refers to the recognition, compilation, and implementation of various methodologies in a comprehensive and inclusive manner. The metaparadigmatic aspect refers to the capacity to weave together, relate, and integrate the various paradigmatic practices.

The paradigmatic aspect refers to all therapies and recovery practices available to and practiced by the client. This is similar to:

> Integral Transformative Practices (ITP), wherein a full range of human potentials are simultaneously engaged and exercised in order to enact and bring forth any higher states and stages of human potential, leading individuals through their own legitimating crisis to an increase in authenticity. (Wilber, 2006, p. 13)

The therapist applies therapies and recommends practices that clients apply and practice that are appropriate for their current recovery altitude and stage of change (DiClemente & Prochaska, 1998). For example, a client in early recovery and at a precontemplation stage of change will be assigned certain practices appropriate for his recovery altitude as well as practices that will help the client to move from a precontemplation to a contemplation stage of change (DiClemente & Prochaska, 1998). The client's recovery altitude and stage of change as well as his or her general stage of development must be considered when choosing appropriate therapies and recovery practices (Wilber, 2006).

The metaparadigmatic aspect refers to its capacity to weave together as well as relate various recovery paradigms to each other. The therapist, by applying integral theory, "generates a meta-practice of honoring, including, and integrating the fundamental paradigms and methodologies of the major forms of human inquiry" (Wilber, 2006, p. 16). From this metaparadigmatic perspective, the therapist acknowledges that all the available recovery-based therapies and recovery practices potentially may have value in their client's recovery when applied at the right time. Furthermore, the therapist is then able to observe how certain therapies and recovery practices relate to and strengthen each other when practiced concurrently. The therapist is then able to orchestrate these recovery paradigms in their client's process.[10] Moreover, the therapist also assists clients to achieve a metaperspective on their own recovery process.

In short, an integrally informed therapist constantly functions from a paradigmatic and metaparadigmatic perspective, therefore, working in an comprehensive and nonexclusive way with his or her clients, while keeping a metaperspective on the interrelatedness and relevance of the recovery paradigms simultaneously in operation in his or her client's process.

CONCLUSION

In this chapter, we explored how the five basic elements of integral theory can inform our understanding of addiction and its treatment. I outlined a tentative proposal for how an integral meta-therapy can be developed, and discussed its paradigmatic and metaparadigmatic features.

In the next chapter, I provide a brief overview of my own application of an integral meta-therapy, called *integrated recovery meta-therapy*.

---

10   What may be useful to develop in the future is a taxonomy of recovery-based interventions, similar to the integral taxonomy of therapeutic interventions (ITTI) as devised by Andre Marquis (2009).

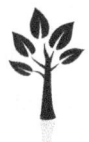

CHAPTER 5

Integrated Recovery Meta-Therapy

Addiction, whatever its form, has always been a desperate search, on a false and hopeless path, for the fulfilment of human freedom.
—MEDARD BOSS (1983, P. 283)

INTRODUCTION

*I*n this chapter, I provide a succinct overview of my own application of an integral meta-therapy, known as integrated recovery meta-therapy (IRMt). IRMt is a meta-therapy in the sense that it provides a big-picture or overarching framework for the therapeutic process with addicted populations.

It is not the aim of the IRMt framework to be specific as to what techniques a therapist must employ, but rather to provide an orienting metaframework of the therapeutic scope and process when working with addicted populations, with the aim that no essential area or process is left out. Yet it must be noted that, as therapists, we are dealing with the immense complexity of another human being that will ultimately remain only partly intelligible to us. The aim of IRMt is simply to make it more intelligible than it would be without a metatheoretical framework, to provide stronger headlights for navigating the recovery journey of a client.

To assist this journey, I have designed visual aids/templates that provide a structure that affords the therapist and client a shared language, and further supplies a way to track progress or lack of progress. It is based on the simple premise that if a recovering addict is engaging in the right practices and developing a recovery-orientated lifestyle then they will likely have a sustainable recovery. It is also important to note IRMt becomes more useful as a meta-therapy once a recovering addict has a stabilized recovery. In short, IRMt is more suitable for those clients that have completed the primary/acute phase of their treatment and for those that acknowledge their addiction and need for a recovery program.

I this chapter, I provide an overview on how to assist a client in compiling an integrated recovery program and to develop a recovery lifestyle. A more detailed discussion of the integrated recovery approach can be found in my book, *An Integral Guide to Recovery: Twelve Steps and Beyond* (Du Plessis, 2015a).[11]

IRMt is principally informed by two philosophical foundations. The first is an existential foundation that defines our being-in-the-world or our recovery-in-the-world, and the second, an overarching metatheoretical foundation informed by integral theory. Although integral theory includes

---

11   A previous version of IRMt was called Integrated Recovery Therapy (Du Plessis, 2012b, 2015), and also included mindfulness-based interventions, positive psychology, and Twelve Step philosophy as part of its theoretical foundation. I have made adjustments to my original approach to keep the foundation metatheoretical, and have not included specific methodological orientations. It is up to the therapist to apply methodology; IRMt merely provides a metatheoretical orientation. It must be added that I view IRMt as open-ended, in the sense that it is a project that is in continuous development, therefore open to incorporate critique and adapt its foundational perspectives.

an existential perspective (among many others), in its metatheoretical orientation, it is important to make the existential foundation of IRMt explicit. I have discussed how to apply integral theory in the context of addiction and recovery in the previous chapter and it is, therefore, unnecessary to discuss it any further. In the next section, I will briefly articulate the existential foundation of IRMt.

EXISTENTIAL FOUNDATION

The term *existential foundation* can be misleading if not defined. In this book, an existential foundation refers to the insights of existential philosophy, existential phenomenology, existential psychology, and existential therapy.[12]

It is beyond the scope of this book to provide a comprehensive discussion of an existential perspective of addiction and recovery, and I will only focus on some aspects that are relevant to IRMt.

In the following section, I briefly explain what these terms mean and how I interpreted them as part of the existential foundation of IRMt. Please note that these are my interpretations of an existential approach to addiction and recovery; other scholars may have significantly different interpretations. Before I proceed in discussing the various influences of the existential foundation of IRMt, I will briefly articulate the importance of an existential foundation for understanding addiction.

Why an Existential Foundation

Most of the models of addiction discussed in the previous chapters have as their foundation a natural scientific worldview and positivistic methodology, which are typically adequate for exploring phenomena that exist on

---

12 The existential foundation that informs IRMt is derived from many existential philosophy and psychology schools of thought, but Medard Boss's approach of Daseinsanalysis is the primary influence.

a certain level of ontological complexity: primarily denoting the physical realm. However, such models are hopelessly inadequate in explaining complex phenomena such as addiction or any human behavior, which exist on higher levels of ontological complexity. For example, reward deficiency syndrome can only be understood as one of many possible physiological risks that interact with other aspects of being human, without having to reduce human behavior and motivation to neurotransmitter levels. Simply put, even though an addict may have altered neurotransmitter levels, concepts such as addiction are meaningless at the molecular realm of brain physiology. To talk at molecular level about addiction is like saying that an amoeba, which only primarily exists in a primitive level of ontological complexity, has abandonment issues originating from poor object relations.

Existential psychiatrist Medard Boss (1983) pointed out that the natural scientific method has its limitations in explaining the human realm as it originated from and is only sovereign in the nonhuman realm (natural sciences). He is of the opinion that "they largely overlook how radically the nature of their object of study—human reality—differs from the make-up of every other realm known to us" (Boss, 1983, p. xxix).[13]

In our current context, one could say that Boss (1983) echoed the dangers of explaining higher-order complex phenomena, for example any aspect of human being-in-the-world, by using methodology (i.e., empirical observation) and epistemology (i.e., positivistic) that are only relevant for lower orders of complexity. He believed that in Freud's metapsychology and most other theories of human existence, there is inevitably an abstraction

---

13 Boss's approach of Daseinsanalysis, based on Heidegger's (1927/1962) ontology, may be edifying in developing a more realistic understanding of addiction. Heidegger developed a method and grounding through which to explore the ontological structure of being human, which he called Dasein; translated as "there-being." Boss's method could be described as an ontic articulation of Heidegger's ontology.

and tapering from our lived engagement in-the-world. In other words, human-being-in-the-world reduced to lower orders of ontic complexity.

Models based on a natural scientific approach, such as biologically oriented models, provide useful information about addiction, but they cannot adequately account for addiction, because human beings are more than their physiology. In fact, the popular brain disease model of addiction, in the light of the above, can only be described as absurd. Boss (1983) suggested that we need an existential philosophical foundation to truly understand what it means to be human and what psychopathology is. An adequate understanding of addiction and recovery should be informed by an existential understanding of human nature, otherwise we remain prone to reducing our being-in-the-world to its constitute parts and consequently, may miss the big picture.

Background

Existential philosophy is often associated with philosophers such as Søren Kierkegaard, Friedrich Nietzsche, Martin Heidegger, and Jean-Paul Sartre. These philosophers dealt with the troubled relationship between man and existence. Kierkegaard (1849/1954) examined his own existence through his existential anxiety, and he found this "angst" has a more potent and drastic reality than any concept. Nietzsche (1883/1954) tried to free man from religious and metaphysical consolations by proclaiming, "God is dead." Heidegger (1927/1962) revolutionized Western ontology by characterizing man as "being-in-the-world" (Dasein), thus, destroying the noted Cartesian aphorism, "I think, therefore I am." Sartre (1943/1971) declared that humans are radically free. Sartre found life to be defined by nothingness, but he believed that man could derive subjective meaning through ownership of one's choices and that man needs a personally meaningful project in order to live.

Existential phenomenology is a form of philosophy that emerged primarily from the combination of existential philosophy and phenomenology. Existentialists and phenomenologists placed special emphasis on man's relational openness with his surroundings (the other). Kierkegaard (1954) indicated that existence

> is a striving, and is both pathetic and comic in the same degree. It is pathetic because the striving is infinite; that is, it is directed toward the infinite [the other], being an actualization of infinitude, a transformation which involves the highest pathos. It is comic, because such a striving involves a self-contradiction. (p. 8)

Husserl (1901/1973) said that our thoughts intentionality, in other words they always refer to something, and are related to objects. It is this openness for the other, in the thought of both existential and phenomenological thinkers, that gave rise to a natural merger between these two schools of thought.

> The central idea of existential philosophy is the concept "existence," which indicates that our being is essentially and always openness to the other. A central idea of phenomenology is that of "intentionality," by which is meant that our consciousness is always consciousness-of-something, i.e., it is interwoven with the other. Precisely because these fundamental ideas are common to existentialism and phenomenology, these two streams of thought have been able to merge into a single stream as existential phenomenology. (Kwant, 1965, p. 23)

By emphasizing the primacy of man as existence or intentionality, existential phenomenologists are interested in the whole man in his relation to the other. Man, as existence or intentionality cannot be reduced to one dimension of his being. He is best understood as existing as the irreducible and inseparable dimensions of feeling, thinking, and acting-in-relation-to-other. Existential man is a whole man that includes the other in his wholeness.

Existential psychology developed at a time when behaviorism and the application of the natural scientific method to psychology and psychotherapy was dominant (May, 1953). The existential psychology approach can be understood as a reaction against this scientific reductionism (studying the parts in an attempt to understand the whole), when trying to understand and describe human behavior and experience.

> Yalom (1980) notes that the scientific tradition has focused too intently on breaking down a complex organism into its parts. These parts, even when combined do not explain the whole. Such research is often found to be inapplicable and inappropriate in explaining the meaning of what the individual is dealing with as it does not focus on the entire subjective experience, rather, on singular aspects of psychic structure (Temple and Gall, 2016, p. 4)

Following the popularity of existential philosophy, existential therapy began to emerge in the 20th century with the work of such thinkers as Ludwig Binswanger, Otto Rank, Medard Boss, Viktor Frankl, Rollo May, Karl Jaspers, and Irvin Yalom (Cooper, 2003).[14] For example, Frankl (1953) drew from his experience in a concentration camp during World War II in formalizing his logotherapy approach, which centers on man's search for meaning. Holding meaninglessness as the central sickness of

---

14   For an excellent introduction to existential psychotherapy see Hans Cohn's (1997) *Existential Thought and Therapeutic Practice: An Introduction to Existential Psychotherapy*. London, England: Sage.

the modern world, Frankl's logotherapy approach centered on man's will to meaning. May (1953) translated key concepts of existential psychology into psychotherapeutic practice, which helped transition the philosophy from Europe to North America. Yalom (1980), who wrote an essential text on existential psychotherapy, centered his existential approach on the four ultimate concerns (derived from the work of Paul Tillich) of clients: death, freedom, existential isolation, and meaninglessness.

Temple and Gall (2016) described the current status of existential therapy by stating that it can be "thought of in four different approaches or schools from which various training programs have emerged" (p. 4). They go on to say that,

> The first school is referred to as Daseinsanalysis, or the analysis of human existence, and is largely influenced by Heidegger's writings (Cooper, 2003b). This approach focuses on an open therapeutic relationship in which the client is able to freely express himself or herself and is moved toward developing openness toward her or his world (Vos et al., 2015). The second school, logotherapy, was developed by Frankl (1992) and aims to help clients discover the meaning and purpose in their lives (Cooper, 2003b, Vos et al., 2015) . . . . The third approach can be identified as the British school of existential psychotherapy and is based largely on the writings of R. D. Laing (Cooper, 2003a; Spinelli, 2007; Vos et al., 2015) and pioneered primarily by Emmy van Deurzen (Cooper, 2003a, Cooper, 2003b). This approach is phenomenological in nature and focuses on exploring the client's experience of existence and relationship with others (Cooper, 2003b; Spinelli, 2007). The final school of thought is often referred to as an American approach and includes the existential–humanistic approach. It focuses primarily on the

client's inward, subjective experience and was established by Rollo May, who acted as mentor to James Bugental, Irving Yalom, and Kirk Schneider (Cooper, 2003a, Cooper, 2003b). From within the American school, two schools have emerged: supportive–expressive group therapy which is directed toward cancer patients; and experiential–existential which focuses on bridging existential therapy with experiential interventions (Vos et al., 2015). (p. 4)

Existential Givens and Existential Anxiety

A central issue in addiction treatment and recovery is how an individual deals with the existential anxiety that arises when confronting ultimate concerns or existential givens. Moreover, addictive behavior can also be understood as a dysfunctional way of dealing with the anxiety induced by a confrontation of existential givens. It is imperative that an individual in recovery finds healthy ways to confront the givens of existence.

There are certain aspects of life that are within our capacity to control and manipulate, but there are also aspects that are given and cannot be avoided; we are "thrown" into these circumstances (Heidegger, 1927/1962). For Yalom (1980), the most significant givens of existence are the unavoidable freedom to choose the way we live our lives, the unavoidability of death, our social isolation, and the meaninglessness of life. For Yalom, the confrontation with these existential givens may evoke anxiety that we often try to circumvent or suppress. What distinguishes existential anxiety from neurotic anxiety, is that all people share the former, it is ontological in nature (Cooper, 2003). Temple and Gall (2016) made the distinction between the concepts of existential anxiety and fear. They point out that:

> Fear is a sensation the individual experiences resulting from an external object, that is, a definitive source. Anxiety, on the other

> hand, has no object, the threat of anxiety is nowhere (Heidegger, 1962; Stolorow, 2007; Tillich, 2000; Weems, Costa, Dehon, & Berman, 2014; Yalom, 1980). For Heidegger (1962), the lack of object in existential anxiety renders external factors meaningless and irrelevant. Existence itself becomes equal to nothingness because embedded in existence is the understanding of the certainty of death, that is, the end of existence. Everyday significance thus collapses and the individual is left with a feeling of strangeness and the sensation of "not-being-at-home" (Heidegger, 1962, p. 188). (p. 7)

In addiction, the existential anxiety generated with a confrontation with these four existential givens is even further magnified. In active addiction, the threat of death is ever present and many addicts have friends that have died as a result of addiction. Addiction isolates the individual in a pursuit that is ultimately meaningless where the capacity to choose is inhibited by the powerlessness over the substance and/or behavior. The experience of meaninglessness has been shown to develop into depression and substance abuse (Moore & Goldner-Vukov, 2009). In the next section, I will focus on one of these existential givens, freedom, and its relation to powerlessness.

Freedom (and Powerlessness)

The concepts of freedom and powerlessness are frequently used in addiction treatment and recovery groups. Freedom is mostly considered a positive state to strive for, and powerlessness as something to be avoided. Yet it is not that simple. Temple and Gall (2016) said that:

> In the existential sense, freedom means to be distinct from external structures however, this leads to being engrossed by dread (Yalom, 1980) or angst (Langdridge, 2013). Human beings desire

structure and experience a sense of being ungrounded when confronted with freedom. (p. 9)

May (1981) believed that freedom can enhance our lives or it can cause one to escape and regress from the "dread" or "angst" that it may bring forth.

Like the existential thinkers, IRMt stresses the significance of freedom, personal responsibility, and freedom of choice. This perspective emphasizes the unique experiences and needs of each individual, and the responsibility each of us has for our choices and what we make of our lives. South African philosopher and statesman Jan Smuts's theory of Holism—in its application to the human personality—is aligned with an existential view of freedom.[15] The striving toward freedom is an essential and central component of Smuts's view of human nature (Du Plessis & Weathers, 2015). Smuts (1926) asserts that:

> To be a free personality represents the highest achievement of which any human being is capable. The Whole is free, and to realize wholeness or freedom (they are orrelative expressions) in the smaller world of individual life represents not only the highest of which the individual is capable, but expresses also what is at once the deepest and highest in the universal movement of Holism. (p. 321)

---

15 Although the concept of holism has been implied by many thinkers, the term *holism*, as academic terminology, was first introduced and appeared publicly in print, by General Jan Smuts (1926) in his book *Holism and Evolution*. He writes that: "Holism (from ὅλος = whole) is the term here coined for this fundamental factor operative towards the creation of wholes in the universe" (p. 86). It must be noted that the concept of holism as introduced and applied by Smuts is not the same as the word "holism" as it is generally applied in many disciplines. Smuts used the word in a metaphysical context, not as a broad principle as it is often used today. Smuts (1926) defined holism as "the ultimate synthetic, ordering, organising, regulative activity in the universe which accounts for all the structural groupings and syntheses in it, from the atom and the physic-chemical structures, through the cell and organisms, through Mind in animals, to Personality in man" (p. 326).

Addiction can be understood as a lifestyle that severely constricts freedom, whereas a recovery lifestyle allows for a fuller expression of freedom and wholeness in our being-in-the-world. A person has the free will to make choices that support either a recovery lifestyle or an addictive lifestyle. The choice and the responsibility is theirs alone. Even though a person might have a condition that limits their free will in relation to their addiction, known as powerlessness in recovery circles, it does not make them powerless over the choices they make, and they have to get the right support and to follow practices that will prevent them from regressing into this powerless condition.

While existential philosophy and psychology applauds the notion of freedom, it also acknowledges limitations of our freedom. The notion of existential limitations has significance in the context of addiction and recovery. From one perspective, addiction can be understood as an attempt to bypass certain of our inherent limitations. While in active addiction, an individual tries to control the uncontrollable, in an attempt to avoid and medicate natural human experiences of pain, disappointment, boredom, and so forth. Ironically, this attempt at control ends up with a person being more out of control, enslaved by the medium which they use to try and control what ultimately cannot be controlled. Flores (1997) pointed out that, "Powerlessness over alcohol and the acceptance of one's limitation in relation to alcohol serves as a prototype for the alcoholic facing and accepting other limitations of the human condition" (p. 273).

Ulman and Paul (2006), in their book *The Self Psychology of Addiction and its Treatment: Narcissus in Wonderland*, brilliantly explained how at the core of addiction dynamics, there is a narcissistic fantasy of having an unrealistic sense of control of oneself, others and things/events in the world:

> In the case of addiction, such a narcissistic fantasy centers on a narcissistic illusion of a megalomaniacal being that possesses magical

control over psychoactive agents (things and activities). These latter entities allow for the artificial alteration of the subjective reality of one's sense of one's self and one's personal world. Under the influence of these intoxicating fantasies, an addict imagines being like a sorcerer or wizard who controls a magic wand capable of manipulating the forces of nature—and particularly the forces of human nature. Eventually, a person becomes a captive of these addictive fantasies and then becomes an addict, lost in a wonderland. (p. 6)

The focus of the next section is how addicts deal with their basic existential needs—either by denying them (trying to control the uncontrollable) or attempting to have these basic existential needs met through destructive or misguided methods.

Basic Existential Needs

Chilean economist, Alfred Max-Neef (1991), who developed the theory of human scale development, stated that:

> Fundamental human needs [basic existential needs] are finite, few and classifiable and are the same in all cultures and in all historical periods. What changes, both over time and through cultures, is the way or the means by which the needs are satisfied. (p. 18)

He went on to say that:

> Each economic, social and political system adopts different methods for the satisfaction of the same fundamental human needs. In every system, they are satisfied (or not satisfied) through the generation (or non-generation) of different types of satisfiers

> [the object or process used to satisfy a need]. We may go as far as to say that one of the aspects that define a culture is its choice of satisfiers. Whether a person belongs to a consumerist or to an ascetic society, his/her fundamental human needs are the same. What changes is his/her choice of the quantity and quality of satisfiers. In short: What is culturally determined are not the fundamental human needs, but the satisfiers for those needs. Cultural change is, among other things, the consequence of dropping traditional satisfiers for the purpose of adopting new or different ones. It must be added that each need can be satisfied at different levels and with different intensities. Furthermore, needs are satisfied within three contexts: (a) with regard to oneself (Eigenwelt); (b) with regard to the social group (Mitwelt); and (c) with regard to the environment (Umwelt). The quality and intensity, not only of the levels but also of contexts, will depend on time, place and circumstances. (p. 18)

According to the theory of human scale development, an individual's quality of life is correlated with the actualization of nine classes of interrelated ontological needs. In this model, needs are categorized in two classes: existential and axiological, which are combined and displayed in a matrix, "This allows us to demonstrate the interaction of, on the one hand, the needs of Being, Having, Doing and Interacting; and, on the other hand, the needs of Subsistence, Protection, Affection, Understanding, Participation, Idleness, Creation, Identity and Freedom" (Max-Neef, 1991, p. 17).

Max-Neef (1991) is of the opinion that:

> Human needs must be understood as a system: that is, all human needs are interrelated and interactive. With the sole exception of

the need of subsistence, that is, to remain alive, no hierarchies exist within the system [as opposed to Maslow's model]. On the contrary, simultaneities, complementarities and trade-offs are characteristics of the process of needs satisfaction. (p. 17)

According to Max-Neef, (1991) any "fundamental human need not adequately satisfied generates a pathology" (p. 22).

In Max-Neef's (1991) model, satisfiers refers to the method of having a basic existential need met (satisfying the need), and various groups of satisfiers are proposed. Five types of satisfiers are suggested: violators or destroyers, pseudo-satisfiers, inhibiting satisfiers, singular satisfiers, and synergic satisfiers. A brief description of each of the types of satisfiers follows. I then conclude with the relevance this has in the context of addiction and its treatment.

Violators or destroyers are paradoxical in nature because when they are applied to satisfy a need, "not only do they annihilate the possibility of its satisfaction over time, but they also impair the adequate satisfaction of other needs" (Max-Neef, 1991, p. 31). Pseudo-satisfiers "generate a false sense of satisfaction of a given need. Although not endowed with the aggressiveness of violators or destroyers, they may on occasion annul, in the not too long term, the possibility of satisfying the need they were originally aimed at fulfilling" (Max-Neef, 1991, p. 31). Inhibiting satisfiers tend to over-satisfy a given need, consequently, limiting the possibility of other needs being satisfied. Singular satisfiers tend to satisfy one specific need. They are neutral in relation to the satisfaction of other needs. Synergic satisfiers satisfy a given need and "simultaneously stimulating and contributing to the fulfillment of other needs" (Max-Neef, 1991, p. 34).

From the above description, it should be clear that addictive behavior can be understood as violators or destroyers, and pseudo-satisfiers. Addictive behavior is always directed at satisfying a need, but what differentiates addictive behavior (violators or destroyers) from other methods (or other satisfiers) of having needs met is that it paradoxically destroys the individual's capacity to meet the need(s) it is attempting to satisfy, as well as the capacity to meet other needs. As an addictive lifestyle progresses, the individual's capacity to have most of his or her needs met is diminished, until there is a near total reliance on the substance or behavior to meet most basic existential needs.

Within the context of the above discussion, it should be clear that a recovery program and lifestyle is a process of replacing destroyers/violators with synergistic and singular satisfiers. A similar sentiment is echoed by Vanhooren, Leijssen, and van Dezutter (2017) in their discussion of the application of experiential and existential approaches to treating criminal offenders:

> Very different from cognitive-behavioral approaches, experiential and existential offender therapies focus on the exploration of the underlying dynamics of criminal behavior in terms of their basic existential needs (Braswell & Wells, 2014; Gunst, 2012; Ronel & Segev, 2014; Vanhooren et al., 2015; Ward & Fortune, 2014). Just like all human beings, offenders try to reach fulfillment of their existential needs, such as the need for efficacy, connectedness, love, and meaning (Braswell & Wells, 2014; Ward & Fortune, 2014). The way they try to fulfill their needs or the way they cope with the inability to reach their goals is often through unadjusted or antisocial behavior (Ward & Fortune, 2014). When the basic existential needs are not met, offenders gradually become stuck in a *criminal spin*: a downward process marked by existential loneliness and alienation (Ronel & Segev, 2014). (p. 15)

An Existential-Phenomenological Perspective of the Twelve Step Program

In the context of our current discussion, and considering the central role that Twelve Step programs have in many addiction treatment centers and programs, it may be useful to explore it from an existential-phenomenological perspective. Moreover, this perspective also highlights some of the reasons why Twelve Step programs are effective.

Carl Thune interpreted AA from a phenomenological perspective and believed one of the reasons AA is effective is because its members share their life histories in AA meetings. He expressed the view that in recounting their life stories, alcoholics are "taught how to interpret their past in a way that gives meaning to the past and hope for the future" (Flores, 1997, p. 281). Thune (1977) wrote about the importance of life histories:

> In a sense, then, one of the first lessons AA must teach new members is that their lives were incoherent and senseless as they knew them. Simultaneously, it must reveal the "correct" understanding and interpretation of the drinking alcoholic's vision of the world before a new member can accept the full benefits of the program—a program which offers a different coherence and meaning to their active alcoholic lives. In other words, according to AA, not only do drinking alcoholics incorrectly perceive and understand the world, but they cannot even correctly perceive and understand their perceptions and understanding of it. Through therapy, they must learn new methods for evaluating them. More abstractly, it is not just a revised and now coherent vision of the world which AA offers, but one which has altered the relation between its components. (pp. 81–82).

AA states that the alcoholic suffers from a spiritually defective mode of being rather than a mere physical disability. For that reason, AA uses a more spiritually-oriented vocabulary "in the absence of a more accurate but inaccessible philosophical-ontological terminology" (Flores, 1997, p. 283). AA believes that alcoholism is only one, albeit the most important, manifestation of a defective lifestyle or mode of being. Stopping drinking, therefore, is the first, but only one aspect of recovery. The alcoholic needs a complete lifestyle change. From a phenomenological perspective, an alcoholic must give up their "self-perceived construction of his or her self that is associated with the alcoholic lifestyle" (Flores, 1997, p. 283). Thune (1977) concluded that "AA's 'treatment,' then involves the systematic manipulation of symbolic elements within an individual's life to provide a new vision of that life and of his world. This provides new coherence, meaning, and implications for behavior" (p. 88).

Another feature of AA that Thune (1977) felt is significant in its success is the constant introduction of oneself as an alcoholic. The self-proclamation of "I am an alcoholic" constantly reminds alcoholics that they are a drink away from their old lives. This is often a problematic issue for those whose interest in AA is superficial or purely academic. Unfortunately, they often fail to see the significance of this ritual. They tend to erroneously equate this statement with a form of self-debasement. What they fail to understand is that alcoholics practice this ritual proudly, and with every introduction, they are indirectly conveying an important message about and to themselves. Flores (1997) stated:

> The term "alcoholic" signifies everything (self-centered behavior, negative attitudes, corrupt values) that sober AA members must guard themselves from if they are to maintain a healthy sobriety. By constantly utilizing the self-definition of alcoholic, AA members

automatically imply the opposite, which is everything a healthy, recovering, and sober member of AA must attain. AA members are thus reminded with each pronouncement of themselves as an alcoholic that they are just a drink away from losing what they have become, which is a person whose values, attitudes, and behavior is the direct opposite of an alcoholic. From this perspective, alcoholism is viewed as more than just excessive drinking. This is why AA believes that alcohol consumption cannot be curtailed without addressing and treating the rest of the alcoholic's personality disturbances. Abstinence from alcohol is the first step required for breaking the alcoholic style of living. (p. 286)

Understanding addiction from this perspective validates the need for a new recovery lifestyle; without a shift in lifestyle and a new set of healthy practices, the addict will eventually gravitate towards his or her habitual mode of being-in-the-world.

Kurtz (1982) is of the opinion that AA works because it shares and addresses many features found in existential philosophy. As mentioned previously, a prominent theme in existential philosophy is the realization that, as humans, we exist within limitations. By admitting their powerlessness over alcohol in Step One, they recognize and admit this fundamental limitation.

Apart from the acceptance of this limitation, AA requires alcoholics to share this limitation with other alcoholics. "The invitation to make such a connection with others and the awareness of the necessity of doing so arise from the alcoholic's very acceptance of limitation" (Kurtz, 1982, p. 53). Although AA suggests the acknowledgment of limitation, it does not abdicate the alcoholic of responsibility. Being confronted by our limitations "engenders the dread, fear, and trembling of Kierkegaard, the angst of Heidegger, the *angoisse* of Sartre, and the abyss of Burber" (Flores, 1997, p. 274).

Furthermore, as indicated previously, a common theme in existential philosophy is the problem of suffering. AA recognizes suffering as an innate aspect of existence, with potential positive influence on our lives. In the context of AA, suffering is given meaning because it creates impetus in the alcoholic to question his or her existence and to be open for change. Viktor Frankl (1953) believed that when we can place our suffering within some meaningful context, we are not defeated by it, but are helped to transcend it.

Similarly, in AA members share "the kinship of suffering" and recovery depends on the mutual sharing of suffering. AA teaches the alcoholic that to be fully human is to need others, and provides alcoholics with a universally shared explanation for their suffering.

From a Buddhist perspective, suffering or *dukkha* is caused by our unwillingness to accept the world as it is and our insistence on trying to make it fit our expected ideas or fantasies. Addiction is, in essence, a refusal to accept things as they are and an attempt to avoid the reality of necessary suffering. An important aspect of recovery is realizing the inevitability of suffering and learning how to cope with it in a healthy way. Happiness is earned only through hard work—not through instant gratification. Flores (1997) summed up this existential predicament of the alcoholic:

> Many existential writers believe that in such a confrontation between the realistic acceptance of the world as it is and the self-centered demands for unlimited gratification, reason would prevail and the individual would choose more realistically between the alternatives—continued unhappy struggles with old patterns of expectations or authentic existence with expanded freedom of choice

and responsible expression of drives and wishes. With Socrates, we argue to 'know thyself.' In this fashion, AA members are taught to believe that the authentic existence advocated by the AA program holds the key to self-examination, self-knowledge, emancipation, cure, and eventual salvation. (p. 280)

THE SIX RECOVERY DIMENSIONS

IRMt views an individual's recovery-in-the-world through six lenses called the recovery dimensions. The six recovery dimensions are influenced by the quadrants of integral theory and Max-Neef's (1991) theory of human scale development. The six recovery dimensions are defined as: physical, which refers to all aspects of physical health; intellectual, which describes all the intellectual features of the recovery process; psychological, which refers to all the emotional and therapeutic aspects; existential, which entails all the spiritual and existential elements; social, which captures all interpersonal, cultural, and social relationships; and environmental, which refers to all administrative, legal, monetary, and environmental aspects (Du Plessis, 2015).[16] Like the quadrants in integral theory, they represent abstract interrelated and nonreducible aspects of our being-in-the-world.

---

16 These six recovery dimensions can be understood as a Quality of Life (QOL) classifications system. QOL is applied as a fundamental concept across health care research (Padaiga, Subata, & Vanagas, 2007), especially in mental health care and disability studies (Masthoff, Trompenaars, Van Heck, Hodiamont, & de Vries, 2005). There has been controversy over the meaning of this concept; no agreement has been reached about its definition (Fischer, Rehm, & Kim, 2001a, 2001b; Moons, Budts, & De Geest, 2006; Taillefer, Dupuis, Roberge, & Le May, 2003). Regardless, QOL is increasingly recognized as a valuable indicator of the impact of treatment, need for health care, evaluation of interventions, and for cost-benefit analyses (Allison, Locker, & Feine, 1997; Foster, Peters, & Marshall, 2000).

116 AN INTEGRAL FOUNDATION FOR ADDICTION TREATMENT

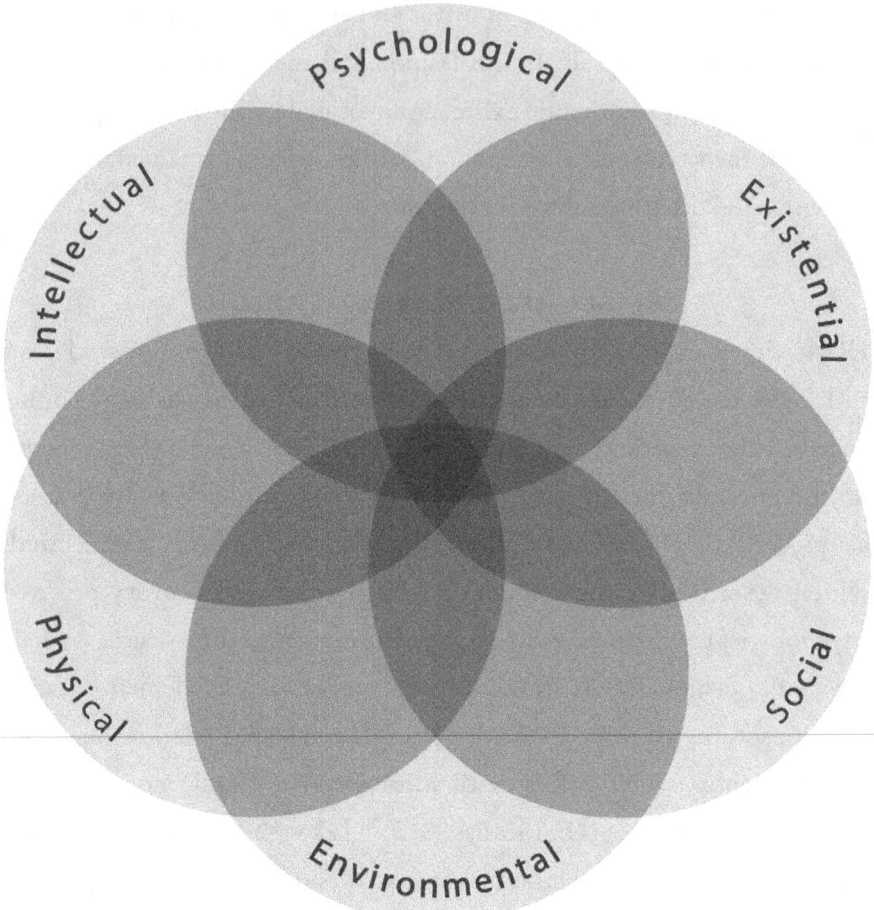

Figure 7: Six Recovery Dimensions[17]

These six interrelated yet irreducible recovery dimensions provide a multiperspectival hexagonal framework on an individual's therapeutic process. According to IRMt, it is vital that these six recovery dimensions of a client are maintained at an essential level of health (what defines essential health is relative and unique for each client) for sustainable recovery. If there

---

17 This image was designed by Guy du Plessis, licensed under the Creative Commons License Attribution-NoDerivs 2.5.

is pathology in any of these areas the whole recovery system suffers (Du Plessis, 2012a, 2015). Clients are assisted by their therapists to find and apply suitable therapies and recovery practices in each of these six recovery dimensions. The therapist works within a continuum of change agents and therefore, does not need to be trained in all the therapies or practices needed in their client's process, but works together with other therapists when necessary, yet always maintains a metaperspective on their client's process. The compilation and action plan of these recovery therapies and practices is defined as the client's integrated recovery program.

The therapist functions like the conductor of an orchestra, keeping a metaperspective of the client's process and ensuring that the various therapies and recovery practices fit together in a balanced way, as well as ensuring that all essential areas of a client's recovery process are addressed.[18] The construct of the six recovery dimensions and the various tools of an integrated recovery program provides an easily accessible recovery structure for both client and therapist that assist in navigating the complex recovery process.

Heidegger (1927/1962) described human existence as being-in-the-world (Dasein). Being-in-the-world encompasses more than human consciousness; it also constitutes the fact that we exist as part of the world. This view points out that we are of the world, rather than in it; we coexist with our world. We and our experience of the world constitute an interdependent unity. A person's existence cannot be reduced to one dimension of his or her being. Rather, his or her existence is best understood as the irreducible and inseparable dimensions of feeling, thinking and acting interdependently

---

18   IRMt is derived from integrated recovery model, originally designed primarily as a clinical model for inpatient treatment protocol design (Du Plessis, 2010), which has shown great promise since its inception and application in 2007 in several Cape Town-based addiction treatment centers. Preliminary research shows promising results (see Duffett, 2010, *Outcomes-based Evaluative Research at an Integrally Informed Substance Abuse Treatment Centre Using the Integrated Recovery Model*).

with others and the world. An existential person is a whole person, who includes others and the world in his or her wholeness.

The different recovery dimensions are informed by this existential view. Each of the recovery dimensions (physical, psychological, intellectual, existential, social, and environmental) constitutes an aspect of our total being-in-the-world; they represent fundamental and irreducible aspects of our existence. When in active addiction, each of these dimensions of an individual's being is affected, and their capacity to authentically exist in the world in each of these dimensions becomes, often severely, limited and dysfunctional. Consequently, for recovery to be sustainable, each of these recovery dimensions needs to be acknowledged as an essential component of a recovery lifestyle.

INTEGRATED RECOVERY PROGRAM

In the following section I will provide a brief outline of the various templates and tools that are used in IRMt: the integrated recovery program template, the integrated recovery wheel, and the integrated recovery indices.

These recovery tools also serve an underlying psychodynamic purpose for recovering addicts. Most addicts suffer from various degrees of pathological narcissism, which can be understood as the regression/fixation to the stage of the archaic, nuclear self. The narcissistically regressed/fixated individual often has a need for omnipotent control, a characteristic of the grandiose self. In active addiction, such power is sought through fusion with an omnipotent self-object (drug of choice) and manifests as impulsivity. Once in recovery, this need for control will initially manifest as the obsessive-compulsive personality traits of ritual and rigidity. Without some clear recovery structure and the absence of the previously idealized self-object (drug/s of choice), the narcissistically regressed individual will be subject to massive anxiety, stemming from fear of fragmentation of self and empty depression, which reflects the scantiness of psychic structure

Chapter 5: Integrated Recovery Meta-Therapy 119

and good internal objects. The structure of an integrated recovery program can help satisfy the need for ritual and rigidity in a healthy way and once this recovery structure is internalized, it will help build much needed psychic structure.

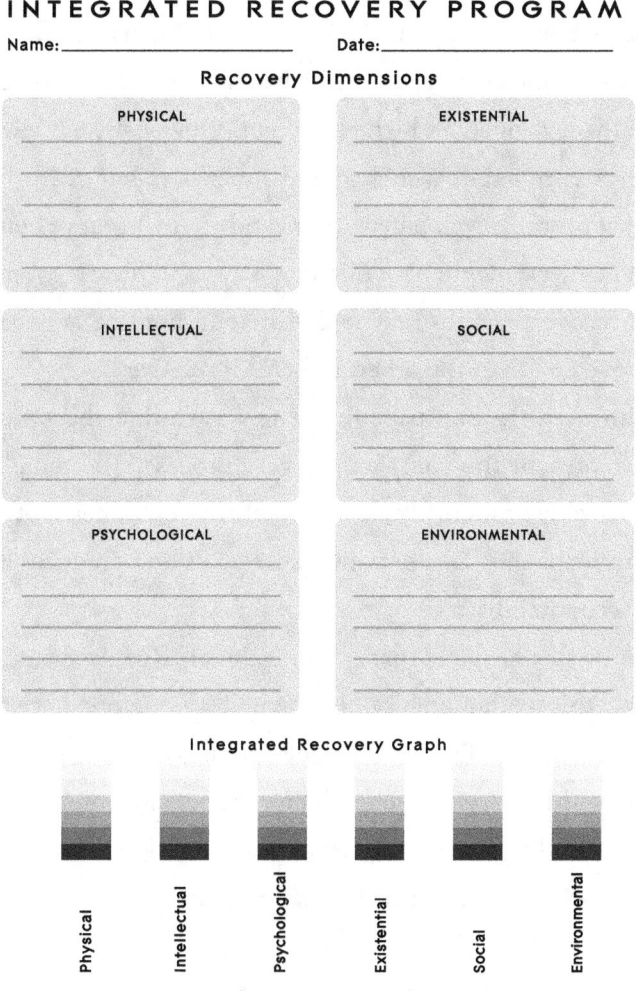

Figure 8: Template for the design of an Integrated Recovery Program (IRP)[19]

---

19 This image was designed by Guy du Plessis, licensed under the Creative Commons License Attribution-NoDerivs 2.5.

An integrated recovery program template provides an outline that an individual in recovery can use to plan his or her personalized integrated recovery program. On the template there are the six recovery dimensions, and the integrated recovery graph.

The integrated recovery graph helps to visually plot the developmental altitude of each of an individual's six recovery dimensions. Therefore, at a glance, therapist and client can see which areas of a client's recovery lifestyle are optimally developed and which are not. Obviously, our clients do not have to be exceptional in each recovery dimension, but rather optimal for their stage of overall development. Somebody with 1 year of being clean or 10 years of being clean will have different focuses in their recovery and their integrated recovery graphs may look different, but one is not necessarily better "recovered" than the other; rather it is relative.

My aim with the one-page template was to find the simplest visual system to represent the complex recovery process. The template can be completed weekly or monthly, or whenever the components of an individual's program change. This provides clear goals and practices as well as a degree of accountability.

It must further be noted that a central aim of IRMt is to teach the client how to apply this method in his or her own life. Therefore, once therapy has been terminated, the client will be able to integrate this metaframework into his or her thinking and doing. Before the second template is discussed, it would be useful to explore the two types of development that happen in a recovery process and how this relates to the templates.

Horizontal/Vertical Development in Recovery

According to Suzanne Cook-Greuter (2004), a leading adult developmental expert, human development can happen vertically (transformation) and horizontally (translation).

> When we talk about development in the context of human development, we distinguish between lateral and vertical development. Both are important, but they occur at different rates. Lateral growth and expansion happens through many channels, such as schooling, training, self-directed and life-long learning as well as simply through exposure to life. Vertical development in adults is much rarer. It refers to how we learn to see the world through new eyes, how we change our interpretations of experience and how we transform our views of reality. It describes increases in what we are aware of, or what we can pay attention to, and therefore what we can influence and integrate. In general, transformations of human consciousness or changes in our view of reality are more powerful than any amount of horizontal growth and learning. (Cook-Greuter, 2004, pp. 2–3)

A therapist can view and measure their client's recovery progress on two planes: the horizontal and vertical, often referred to as translating and transformation in integral psychology (Forman, 2010; Ingersoll & Zeitler, 2010). Clients' vertical growth in recovery refers to how they grow developmentally—here we can use various developmental models (Cook-Greuter, 2004; Wilber, 2000). As clients slowly and painstakingly grow through these vertical stages, their perspective of themselves and the world changes: it gradually becomes less self-centered, more inclusive, and embracing (Wilber, 2000).

Horizontal development indicates how well a client is applying their recovery tools at a certain stage of development and how well they are integrated at that stage. This is far more important than aiming for the next stage of development. The idea is that working a recovery program eventually translates into vertical development or transformation. One of the primary aims of a recovery therapist is to help clients translate effectively at their current stages of development and not just aim at vertical growth.

Clients use the integrated recovery graph to indicate their vertical development in each of the recovery dimensions. As we have seen, each of the six recovery dimensions can also be at different stages of vertical development. For the sake of simplicity, the integrated recovery graph plots three stages: pathological, adequate, and excellent.

The horizontal or lateral growth of a client indicates how well they have practiced each of their recovery dimensions within a chosen time frame, which could be daily, weekly, or even monthly. The scales used for horizontal growth do not correlate with stages of development, but can be compared with a test or assessment of a practice, as in, "How much of what you should have done did you do?" The idea is that constant horizontal practice (or translation) in a recovery dimension will translate into vertical development (or transformation) in that recovery dimension, and eventually contribute to overall vertical development.

I apply a hexagonal-circular model called the integrated recovery wheel to illustrate a recovery lifestyle on a horizontal plane and within a chosen time frame. The inner circle signals dangerous behaviors or risk factors and the outer circle signifies the healthy practices or protective factors that are taking place in the six recovery dimensions within a specific time frame.

From a needs perspective, the outside circle represents healthy ways of having needs met (Singular or Synergistic Satisfiers). On the other hand, the inner circle represents unhealthy attempts of having your needs met, pseudo-satisfiers "that generate a false sense of satisfaction of a given need" (Max-Neef, 1991, p. 31).

Chapter 5: Integrated Recovery Meta-Therapy

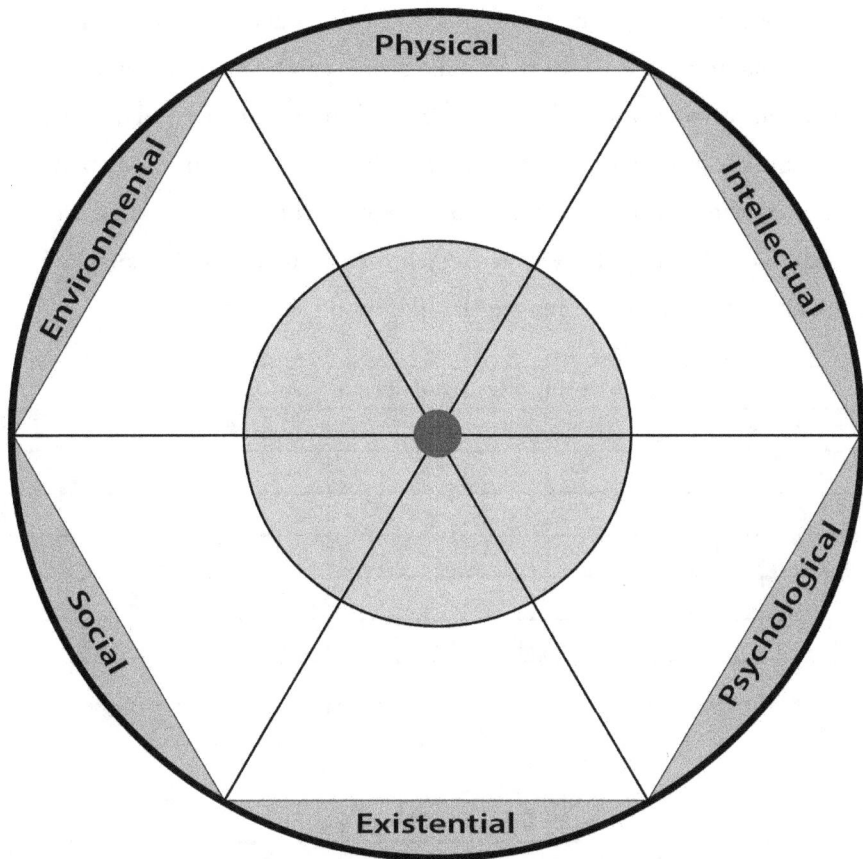

Figure 9: The Integrated Recovery Wheel[20]

The integrated recovery wheel is used in the form of a daily diary, where, for each of the six recovery dimensions, healthy recovery actions (protective factors) are indicated in the outer circle and dangerous behaviors (risk factors) are indicated in the center. Each day, clients can also score themselves (from 0 to 10) for each of their recovery dimensions. This provides them with a total daily score when added together as well as a weekly score for each recovery dimension when the scores for each day in the week are totaled.

---

20 This image was designed by Guy du Plessis, licensed under the Creative Commons License Attribution-NoDerivs 2.5.

For the purpose of keeping scores of their horizontal development, they can use various indices. Each of their daily scores can be recorded on a weekly integrated recovery index for each week and then over a period of a month on a monthly integrated recovery index. These enable them to see patterns in the way they practice their recovery program. If they continue on average to score well in each of their recovery dimensions, this will translate into vertical development and reduce the likelihood of relapse.

Monthly Integrated Recovery Index							
	Week 1	Week 2	Week 3	Week 4	Week 5		Total:
Phys							
Intel							
Psych							
Exis							
Soc							
Env							

Weekly Integrated Recovery Index									
	Mon	Tues	Wed	Thurs	Fri	Sat	Sun		Total:
Phys									
Intel									
Psych									
Exis									
Soc									
Env									
								Total:	

Figure 10: Integrated Recovery Indices[21]

---

21   This image was designed by Guy du Plessis, licensed under the Creative Commons License Attribution-NoDerivs 2.5.

Chapter 5: Integrated Recovery Meta-Therapy

BEING-IN-RECOVERY AND DOING-IN-RECOVERY

One of the perils of any personal development program is that we can develop unrealistic expectations of ourselves and our development. Unrealistic expectations force us to continuously measure ourselves against unattainable and perfectionist ideals. Instead of improving our well-being, this adds to our distress and feelings of inadequacy.

Recovering addicts working in a recovery program run the risk of succumbing to this inherent problem. Addicts are known to have perfectionistic tendencies with overdeveloped inner critics, fueled by low self-esteem an internalized shame. Their low self-esteem often drives them relentlessly to prove to themselves and others that they are good enough.

Throughout most of this chapter, I have focused primarily on the doing of recovery, the practice components of a recovery lifestyle. Another equally important, and perhaps even more important component of recovery, is what I call the "modes of being-in-recovery." What I mean by this term is that for every recovery practice, there is an attitudinal, or being, component, which is the way we relate to the practice. These modes of being-in-recovery can positively or negatively influence the outcome of a person's recovery practices.

The practice, or doing-in-recovery, should not be confused with being-in-recovery. Very often, those of who are involved in a process of self-development or a recovery program spend so much time practicing and self-developing that they forget to live; forget to enjoy just being and being-with-others.

The attitude of participation will affect the value one gets from the practice. I call these attitudinal or modes of being-in-recovery our "existential attitude" toward a practice. In short, each recovery practice can be understood as having two qualities: the doing or the result of the practice, and the being or existential attitude toward the practice. Each recovery dimension may consist of healthy practices, which are done to the utmost, but if they are done with an undesirable existential attitude, it will seriously compromise or could even have a destructive effect on a client's well-being. For example, a client could be going to gym five times a week, but if this is mediated by existential attitudes, like perfectionism and over-criticalness, it could result in a negative influence on his or her recovery.

I would go as far to say that the overall quality of an individual's recovery is determined by the quality of their existential attitudes, rather than the results of their practices. In practical terms, this means that when clients design their programs, they (and we as therapists) should remain mindful of the existential attitudes mediating these practices.

In conclusion, it is important that your clients maintain a healthy balance between doing and being, and that their recovery program does not become another futile attempt (like their substance use and addictive behavior) to "fix what ain't broke." Recovery practice is a paradox. Individuals in recovery have to work hard, not to be better, but merely to become conscious of the fact that essentially they are good enough as they are right now. The ultimate aim of working a recovery program is not about being fixed, but rather the slow process of realizing that there is nothing to fix.

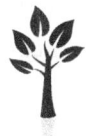

CONCLUSION

In the last resort a civilization depends on its general ideas; it is nothing but a spiritual structure of the dominant ideas expressing themselves in institutions and the subtle atmosphere of culture. If the soul of our civilization is to be saved we shall have to find new and fuller expression for the great saving unities—the unity of reality in all its range, the unity of life in all its forms, the unity of ideas throughout human civilization, and the unity of man's spirit with the mystery of the Cosmos in religious faith and aspiration.
—GENERAL JAN SMUTS (1926, PP. V-VI)

*I*n the previous chapters it was pointed out that the two foremost problems in the field of addiction science and addiction treatment are definitional confusion (Shaffer et al., 2004; Vaillant, 1995; White, 1998) and the ineffectiveness of treatment (Alexander, 2010; Fields, 1998; Hill, 2010; Shaffer, 1997; Shaffer et al., 2004; White, 1998). Many scholars agree that a paradigm shift is urgently needed for the field of addiction because currently, there is such an abundance and diversity of addiction theories

(Hill, 2010; Shaffer, 1997; Shaffer et al., 2004; Vaillant; 1995; White, 1998) that the field of addictionology is in conceptual chaos.

It was argued that the development of an alternative ontological foundation for addiction could possibly assist moving toward conceptual integration and improving treatment outcomes. In this book, it was proposed that integral theory could provide this much-needed alternative ontological (as well as epistemological and methodological) foundation for addiction.

Various elements of integral theory's postmetaphysical position was explored, and although the argument presented in this book has several limitations, it can be concluded that integral theory has great potential as a framework for conceptual integration in addiction studies and improving treatment outcomes, and warrants further research and exploration.[22]

Only a truly integral approach may be able to adequately address the massive and mind-boggling, complex problem of addiction. As the great philosopher-statesman, Jan Smuts (1926,) declared: "If the soul of our civilization is to be saved we shall have to find new and fuller expression for the great saving unities" (p. vi). This book has indicated that integral theory could serve as a "fuller expression" in the quest for a comprehensive understanding of addiction, and as a result—beyond the realm of theories and academia—can help save lives.

---

22 My current research is exploring the relationship between ideology and addiction from an integral perspective. I propose that ideologies are psychoactive and potentially addictive. Ideology addiction can be understood as a type of ideological possession and zealotry, with deleterious consequences for the individual and society. An individual in the grips of an ideology addiction exhibits psychological and behavioral patterns common to all addicted populations. From a psychodynamic perspective, ideology addiction can be understood as the result of a narcissistic disturbance of self experience and deficits in self capabilities. Consequently, the activism of an ideology addict is fundamentally a narcissistic project. A misguided attempt at self repair and satisfaction of archaic narcissistic needs, and seldom motivated by the ideals of the ideology.

REFERENCES

Adesso, V. J. (1985). Cognitive factors in alcohol and drug abuse. In M. Galizio & S. A. Maisto (Eds.), *Determinates of substance abuse: Biological, psychological, and environmental factors* (pp. 125–178). New York, NY: Plenum Press.

Alcoholics Anonymous. (1987). *Twelve steps and twelve traditions.* New York, NY: AA World Services.

Alexander, B. K. (2008). *The globalization of addiction: A study in poverty of the spirit.* Oxford, England: Oxford University Press.

Alexander, B. K. (2010). A change of venue for addiction. Retrieved from http://www.brucekalexander.com/articles-speeches/176-change-of-venue-1

Allison, P. J., Locker, D., & Feine, J. S. (1997). Quality of life: A dynamic construct. *Social Science & Medicine, 45,* 221–230.

Amodia, D. S., Cano, C., & Eliason, M. J. (2005). An integral approach to substance abuse. *Journal of Psychoactive Drugs, 37,* 363–371.

Bandura, A. (1977). *Social learning theory.* Englewood Cliffs, NJ: Prentice-Hall.

Bandura, A. (1986) *Social foundations of thoughts and action: A social cognitive theory.* Englewood Cliffs, NJ: Prentice-Hall.

Barrett. R. J. (1985). Behavioral approaches to individuals' differences in substance abuse. Drug-taking behavior. In M. Galizio & S. A. Maisto (Eds.), *Determinates of substance abuse: Biological, psychological, and environmental factors* (pp. 125–178). New York, NY: Plenum Press.

Batson, H., Brown, L. S., Jr., Zaballero, A., & Faulcon-Gary, J. (1992). A multicomponent model for substance abuse treatment. *Journal of Substance Abuse Treatment, 9*(2), 177–181.

Begleiter, H., & Porjesz, B. (1999). What is inherited in the predisposition toward alcoholism? A proposed model. *Alcoholism: Clinical and Experimental Research, 23*, 1125–1135.

Bishop, R. C. (2007). *The philosophy of the social sciences: An introduction.* London, England: Continuum.

Blomqvist, J., & Cameron, D. (2002). Moving away from addiction: Forces, processes and contexts. *Addiction Research and Theory 10*, 115–118.

Blum, K. (1995, April). Reward deficiency syndrome: Electro-physiological and biogenetic evidence. Paper presented at the annual meeting of the Society for the Study of Neuronal Regulation, Scottsdale, AZ.

Blume W. A. (2004), Understanding and diagnosing substance use disorder. In R. H. Coombs (Ed.), *Handbook of addictive disorders: A practical guide to diagnosis and treatment* (pp. 63–93). Hoboken. NJ: John Wiley & Sons.

Bohman, J. (1993). *New philosophy of social science: Problems of indeterminacy.* Cambridge, MA: MIT Press.

Boss, M. (1983). *The existential foundations of medicine and psychology.* New York, NY: Jason Aronson.

Bowden, J., & Gravitz, H. (1998) *Genesis: Spirituality in recovery from childhood traumas.* Deerfield Beach, FL: Health Communications.

Brick, J., & Erickson, C. (1999). *Drugs, the brain, and behavior: The pharmacology of abuse and dependence.* New York, NY: Haworth Medical Press.

Brodie, J. F., & Redfield, M. (2002). *High anxieties: Cultural studies in addiction.* Berkeley, CA: University of California Press.

Brown, S. A. (1993). Recovery patterns in adolescent substance abuse. In J. S. Baer, G. A. Marlatt, & R. J. McMahon (Eds.), *Addictive behaviors across the lifespan: Prevention, treatment and policy issues* (pp. 161–183). Newbury Park, CA: Sage.

Califano, J. (2008). *High society: How substance abuse ravishes America and what to do about it.* New York, NY: Perseus Books.

Campbell, R. J. (1996). *Psychiatric dictionary* (7th ed.). New York, NY: Oxford Press.

Cappell, H., & Greeley, J. (1987). Alcohol and tension reduction: An update on research and theory. In H. T. Blane & K. E. Leonard (Eds.), *Psychological theories of drinking and alcoholism* (pp. 15–89). New York, NY: Guilford Press.

Carnes, P. (2008). *Recovery start kit.* Carefree, AZ: Gentle Path Press.

Chassin L., Patrick, C. J., Andrea, H. M., & Craig, C. R. (1996). The relations of parent alcoholism to adolescent substance use: A longitudinal follow-up study. *Journal of Abnormal Psychology, 105,* 70–80.

Coleman, B. S. (1980). Incomplete mourning and addict/family transactions: A theory for understanding heroin abuse. In D. J. Lettieri, M. Sayers, H. W. Pearson (Eds.), *Theories on drug abuse: Selected contemporary perspectives* (NIDA Monograph No. 30; pp. 83–89). Washington, DC: Government Printing Office.

Connors, G. J., & Tarbox, A. R. (1985). Macroenvironmental factor determinants of substance use and abuse. In M. Galizio & S. A. Maisto (Eds.), *Determinants of substance abuse: Biological, psychological, and environmental factors* (pp. 283–314). New York, NY: Plenum Press.

Cook-Greuter, S. (2004). Making the case for a developmental perspective. *Industrial and Commercial Training, 36*(7), 275–281.

Cooper, M. (2003). *Existential therapies.* London, England: Sage.

Coppelo, A., & Orford, J. (2002), Addiction and the family: Is it time for services to take notice of the evidence? *Addiction, 97*, 1361–1363.

Corey, G. (2005). *Theory and practice of counselling and psychotherapy.* (7th ed). Pacific Grove, CA: Brooks Cole.

Dawson, D. A., Grant, B. F., Stinson F. S., & Chou, D. S. (2006). Estimating the effect of help seeking on achieving recovery from alcohol dependence. *Addiction, 101*, 824–834.

Dewey, J. (1981). *The philosophy of John Dewey.* Ed. J. McDermott. Chicago: University of Chicago Press.

DiClemente, C. C. (2003). *Addiction and change: How addictions develop and addicted people recover.* New York, NY: Guilford Press.

DiClemente, C. C., & Prochaska, J. O. (1998). Toward a comprehensive, transtheoretical model of change: Stages of change and addictive behaviours. In W. R. Miller & N. Heather (Eds.), *Treating addictive behaviours* (2nd ed., pp. 3–24). New York, NY: Plenum Press.

Donovan, D. M., & Marlatt, G. A. (Eds). (1998). *Assessment of addictive behaviours.* New York, NY: Guilford Press.

Duffett, L. (2010). Outcomes-based evaluative research at an integrally informed substance abuse treatment centre using the Integrated Recovery model (Unpublished thesis). University of Cape Town, South Africa.

Du Plessis, G. P. (2010). The integrated recovery model for addiction treatment and recovery. *Journal of Integral Theory and Practice, 5*(3), 68–87.

Du Plessis, G. P. (2012a). Integrated recovery therapy: Toward an integrally informed individual psychotherapy for addicted populations. *Journal of Integral Theory and Practice, 7*(1), 124–148.

Du Plessis, G. P. (2012b). Toward an integral model of addiction: By means of integral methodological pluralism as a metatheoretical and integrative conceptual framework. *Journal of Integral Theory and Practice, 7*(3), 1–24.

Du Plessis, G. P. (2013, July) *The import of integral pluralism in striving towards an integral metatheory of addiction*. Paper presented at the Third Biennial Integral Theory Conference, San Francisco, CA.

Du Plessis, G. P. (2014a). An integral ontology of addiction: A multiple object existing as a continuum of ontological complexity. *Journal of Integral Theory and Practice, 9*(1), 38–54.

Du Plessis, G. P. (2014b). *Towards an integral meta-theory of addiction* (Master's dissertation, University of South Africa, Pretoria, South Africa.

Du Plessis, G. P. (2015) *An integral guide to recovery: Twelve steps and beyond*. Tuscon, AZ: Integral Publishers.

Du Plessis, G. P., & Weathers, B. (2015, July). *The integral Jan Smuts*. Paper presented at the Fourth International Integral Theory Conference, San Francisco, CA.

Dupuy, J., & Gorman, A. (2010). Integral recovery: An AQAL approach to inpatient alchohol and drug treatment. *Journal of Integral Theory and Practice, 5*(3), 86–101.

Dupuy, J., & Morelli, M. (2007). Toward an integral recovery model for drug and alcohol addiction. *Journal of Integral Theory and Practice, 2*(3), 26–42.

Edwards, M. G. (2008a). Evaluating integral metatheory. *Journal of Integral Theory and Practice, 3*(4), 61–83.

Edwards, M. G. (2008b). Where's the method to our integral madness? An outline of an integral meta-studies. *Journal of Integral Theory and Practice, 3*(2), 165–194.

Edwards, M. G. (2010). *Organizational transformation for sustainability: An integral metatheory*. New York, NY: Routledge.

Edwards, M. G. (2013). Towards an integral meta-studies: Describing and transcending boundaries in the development of big picture science. *Integral Review, 9*(2), 173–188.

Engel, G. L. (1977). The need for a new medical model. *Science, 196*, 129–136.

Engel, G. L. (1980). The clinical applications of the biopsychosocial model. *American Journal of Psychiatry, 5*, 535–544.

Erickson, C. K. (1989). Reviews and comments on alcohol research relaxation therapy, and endorphins in alcoholics. *Alcoholism, 6*, 525–526.

Esbjörn-Hargens, S. (2006). Integral research: A multi-method approach to investigating phenomena. *Constructivism and the Human Sciences, 11*(1), 79–107.

Esbjörn-Hargens, S. (2009). An overview of integral theory: An all-inclusive framework for the 21st century (Resource Paper No. 1). Boulder, CO: Integral Institute.

Esbjörn-Hargens, S. (2010). An ontology of climate change. *Journal of Integral Theory and Practice, 5*(1), 143–174.

Esbjörn-Hargens, S., & Zimmerman. M. E. (2009). *Integral ecology: Uniting multiple perspectives on the natural world.* New York, NY: Integral Books.

Fischer, B., Rehm, J., & Kim, G. (2001a). Quality of Life (QoL) in illicit drug addiction treatment and research: Concepts, evidence and questions. In B. Westermann, C. Jellinek, & G. Belleman (Eds.), *Substitution: Zwischen Leben und Sterben* (pp. 21–40). Weilheim, Germany: Beltz Deutscher Studien Verlag.

Fischer, B., Rehm, J., & Kim, G. (2001b). Whose quality of life is it, really? *British Medical Journal, 322*, 1357–1360.

Flores, P. J. (1997). *Group psychotherapy with addicted populations.* Binghamton, NY: The Haworth Press.

Forman, M. (2010) *A guide to integral psychotherapy: Complexity, integration and spirituality in practice.* New York, NY: SUNY Press.

Foster, J. H., Peters, T. J., & Marshall, E. J. (2000). Quality of life measures and outcome in alcohol-dependent men and women. *Alcohol, 22*, 45–52.

Frankl, V. (1953). *Man's search for meaning.* Boston, MA: Beacon.

Gardner, H. (1983). *Frames of mind*. New York, NY: Basic Books.

Gifford, E., & Humphreys, K. (2006). The psychological science of addiction. *Addiction and its Sciences, 102*, 352–361.

Glantz, M., & Pickens, R. (Eds.). (1992). *Vulnerability to drug abuse*. Washington, DC: American Psychological Association.

Gorman, A. (2013), *Integral recovery: A case study of an AQAL [all-quadrants, all-levels, all-lines, all-states, all-types] approach to addiction treatment* (Doctoral dissertation). John F. Kennedy University, Pleasant Hill, CA.

Gordis, E. (2000). From genes to geography: The cutting edge of alcohol research. *Alcohol Alert, 48*. Rockville MD: National Institute of Alcohol and Drug Abuse.

Graham, M. D., Young, R. A., Valach, L., & Wood, R. A. (2008). Addiction as a complex social action: An action theoretical perspective. *Addiction Research and Theory, 16*, 121–133.

Griffiths, M. D. (2005). A components model of addiction within a biopsychosocial framework. *Journal of Substance Use, 10*, 191–197.

Griffiths, M. D., & Larkin, M. (2004). Conceptualizing addiction: A case for a complex systems account. *Addiction Research and Theory, 12*, 99–102.

Grof, S. (1980). *LSD psychotherapy*. Pomona, CA: Hunter House.

Grof, S. (1992). *The holotropic mind*. San Francisco, CA: Harper Collins.

Gruber, H. E., & Voneche, J. J. (Eds.). (1977). *The essential Piaget*. New York, NY: Basic Books.

Hampson, G. P. (2007). Integral re-views postmodernism: The way out is through. *Integral Review, 4*, 108–173.

Hawkins, J. D., Catalano, R. F., & Miller, J. Y. (1994). Risk and protective factors for alcohol and other drug problems in adolescence and early adulthood: Implications for substance use prevention. *Psychological Bulletin, 112*, 64–105.

Heidegger, M. (1962). *Being and time* (J. Macquarrie & E. Robinson, Trans.). New York, NY: Harper. (Original work published 1927)

Hesselbrock, M. N., Hesselbrock, V. M., & Epstein, E. E. (1999). Theories of etiology of alcohol and other drug disorders. In B. S. McCrady & E. E. Epstein (Eds.), *Addictions: A comprehensive guidebook* (pp. 50–74). New York, NY: Oxford University Press.

Hill, W. B. (2010). *An ontological analysis of mainstream addiction theories: Exploring relational alternatives* (Doctoral dissertation). Retrieved from ProQuest Dissertations and Theses database. (UMI No. 3402363)

Hinson, R. E. (1985). Individual differences in tolerance and relapse: A Pavlovian conditioning perspective. In M. Galizio & S. A. Maisto (Eds.), *Determinates of substance abuse: Biological, psychological and environmental factors* (pp. 125–178). New York, NY: Plenum Press.

Hoffman, R. S., & Goldfrank, L. R. (1990). The impact of drug abuse and addiction on society. *Emergency Medicine Clinics of North America. 8*, 469–480.

Holford, P., Miller, D., & Braly, J. (2008). *How to quit without feeling s**t*. London, England: Piatkus Books.

Husserl, E. (1901/1973). *Logical Investigations*. Trans. J. N. Findlay, London: Routledge.

Ingersoll, R. E., & Zeitler, D. M. (2010) *Integral psychotherapy: Inside out/ Outside in*. New York, NY: SUNY Press.

Jay, J., & Jay, D. (2000). *First love: A new approach to intervention for alcoholism and drug addiction*. Center City, MN: Hazelden.

Jessor, R., & Jessor, S. L. (1977). *Problem behavior and psychosocial development*. New York, NY: Academic Press.

Jessor, R., & Jessor, S. (1980). A social-psychological framework for studying drug use. In In D. J. Lettieri, M. Sayers, & H. W. Persons (Eds.),

Theories on drug abuse: Contemporary perspectives (NIDA Research Monograph No. 30; pp. 102–109). Washington, DC: U.S. Government Printing Office.

Johnson, D. B. (1980). *Toward a theory of drug subcultures.* Rockville, MD: National Institute on Drug Abuse.

Jung, J. (2001). *Psychology of alcohol and other drugs: A research perspective.* Thousand Oaks. CA: Sage.

Kandel, D. B., & Davies, M. (1992). Progression to regular marijuana involvement: Phenomenology and risk factors for near daily use. In M. Glantz & R. Pickens (Eds.), *Vulnerability to drug abuse* (pp. 299–358). Washington, DC: American Psychological Association.

Kernberg, O. F. (1975). *Borderline conditions and pathological narcissism.* New York, NY: Jason Aroson.

Khantzian, E. J. (1999). *Treating addiction as a human process.* Northvale, NJ: Jason Aronson.

Khantzian, E. J., Halliday, K. S., & McAuliffe, W. E. (1990). *Addiction and the vulnerable self: Modified dynamic group therapy for substance abusers.* New York, NY: Guilford Press.

Kierkegaard, S. (1954). *The sickness unto death.* New York, NY: Doubleday. (Original work published 1849)

Kinney, J. (2003). *Loosening the grip: A handbook of alcohol information.* (7th ed.). New York, NY: McGraw-Hill.

Kohut, H. (1971). *The analysis of the self: A systematic approach to the psychoanalytic treatment of narcissistic personality disorders.* New York, NY: International University Press.

Kohut, H. (1977). *The restoration of self.* New York, NY: International University Press.

Kurtz, E. (1979). *Not-God: A history of Alchoholics Anonymouse.* Center City, MN: Hazeldon.

Kurtz, E. (1982). Why AA works: The intellectual significance of Alcoholics Anonymous. *Quarterly Journal of Studies on Alcohol, 43*, 38–80.

Kurtz, E., & Ketcham, K. (2002). *The spirituality of imperfection: Storytelling and the search for meaning.* New York, NY: Bantam Books.

Laffaye, C., McKellar, J. D., Ilgen, M. A., & Moos, R. H. (2008). Predictors of 4-year outcome of community residential treatment for patients with substance use disorders. *Addictions, 103*, 670–680.

Laudet, A. B., Morgen, K., & White, W. L. (2006). The role of social supports, spirituality, religiousness, life meaning and affiliation with 12-Step fellowship in quality of life satisfaction among individuals in recovery from alcohol and drug problems. *Alcoholism Treatment Quarterly, 24*(1–2), 33–73.

Levant, R. F. (2004). 21st century psychology: Toward a biopsychosocial model. *Psychotherapy Bulletin, 39*(2), 8–11.

Levin, J. D. (1995). Psychodynamic treatment of alcohol abuse. In J. P. Barber & P. Crits-Christoph (Eds.), *Dynamic therapies for psychiatric disorders: Axis 1* (pp. 193–229). New York, NY: Basic Books.

Lewis, M. W., & Kelemen, M. L. (2002). Multiparadigm inquiry: Exploring organizational pluralism and paradox. *Human Relations, 55*(2), 251–275.

Marlatt, G. A., & Gordon, J. R. (1985). *Relapse prevention: Maintenance strategies in treatment of addictive behaviors.* New York, NY: Guilford Press.

Martin, J. A. (2008). Integral research as a practical mixed-methods framework: Clarifying the role of integral methodological pluralism. *Journal of Integral Theory and Practice, 3*(2), 155–164.

Marquis, A. (2008). *The integral intake: A comprehensive idiographic assessment in integral psychotherapy.* New York, NY: Taylor & Francis.

Marquis, A. (2009). An integral taxonomy of therapeutic interventions. *Journal of Integral Theory and Practice, 4*(2), 13–42.

Masthoff, E., Trompenaars, F., Van Heck, G., Hodiamont, P., & De Vries, J. (2005). Validation of the WHO Quality of Life assessment instrument (WHOQOL-100) in a population of Dutch adult psychiatric outpatients. *European Psychiatry, 20*, 465–473.

Max-Neef, M. A. (with Antonio, E., & Hopenhayn, M.). (1991). *Human scale development: Conception, application and further reflections.* New York, NY: Apex.

May, R. (1953). *Man's search for himself.* New York, NY: Dell.

May, R. (1981). *Freedom and destiny.* New York, NY: W. W. Norton.

McPeak, J. D., Kennedy, B. P., & Gordon, S. M. (1991). Altered states of consciousness therapy: A missing component in alcohol and drug rehabilitation treatment. *Journal of Substance Abuse Treatment, 8*, 75–82.

Meehl, P. (1992). Cliometric metatheory: The actuarial approach to empirical, history-based philosophy of science. *Psychological Reports, 71*(2), 339–467.

Meissner, W. W. (1980). Addiction and paranoid process: Psychoanalytic perspectives. *International Journal of Psychoanalytic Psychotherapy, 8*, 273–310.

Menninger, K. A. (1938). *Man against himself.* New York, NY: Harcourt & Brace.

Merikangas, K. R., Rounsaville, B. J., & Prusoff, B. A. (1992). Familial factors in vulnerability to drug abuse. In M. Glantz & R. Pickens (Eds.), *Vulnerability to drug abuse* (pp. 75–97). Washington, DC: American Psychological Association.

Milkman, H. B., & Sunderworth, S. G. (2010). *Craving for ecstasy and natural highs: A positive approach to mood alteration.* Thousand Oaks, CA: Sage.

Miller R. W. (1997). Spiritual aspects of addiction treatment and research. *Mind/Body Medicine, 2*(1), 37–43.

Miller, R. W. (1998). Researching the spiritual dimensions of alcohol and other drug problems. *Addiction, 93*(7), 979–990.

Miller, W. R. (2006). Motivational factors in addictive behaviors. In W. R. Miller & K. M. Carroll (Eds.), *Rethinking substance abuse: What the science shows, and what we should do about it* (pp. 134–152). New York, NY: Guilford Press.

Miller, W. R., & Carroll, K. M. (2006). Drawing the scene together: Ten principles, ten recommendations. In W. R. Miller & K. M. Carroll (Eds.), *Rethinking substance abuse: What the science shows, and what we should do about it* (pp. 293–312). New York, NY: Guilford Press.

Miller, W. R. & Rollnick, S. (2002). *Motivational interviewing: Preparing people to change*. New York, NY: Guilford Press.

Moons, P., Budts, W., & De Geest, S. (2006). Critique on the conceptualisation of quality of life: A review and evaluation of different conceptual approaches. *International Journal of Nursing Studies, 43*, 891–901.

Moore, L. J., & Goldner-Vukov, M. (2009). The existential way to recovery. *Psychiatra Danubina, 21*, 453–462.

Moos, H. R. (2003). Addictive disorders in context: Principles and puzzles of effective treatment and recovery. *Psychology of Addictive Behaviors,17*, 3–12.

Murray, T. (2010). Exploring epistemic wisdom: Ethical and practical implications of integral theory and methodological pluralism for collaboration and knowledge-building. In S. Esbjörn-Hargens (Ed.), *Integral theory in action: Applied, theoretical, and constructive perspectives on the AQAL model* (pp. 345–367). Albany, NY: Suny Press.

Murray, T. (2011). Toward post-metaphysical enactments: On epistemic drives, negative capability, and indeterminacy analysis. *Integral Review, (7)*2, 92–125.

Murray, T. (2012). Embodied realisms and integral ontologies: Towards self-critical theories. Retrieved from http://www.perspegrity.com/papers/Murray_Metaphorical_Realisms.pdf

Myers, B., & Parry, C. (2004). Access to substance abuse treatment services for black South Africans: Findings from audits of specialist treatment facilities in Cape Town and Gauteng. *South Africa Psychiatry Review, 8,* 15–19.

Nakken, C. M. (1998). *Understanding the addictive process: Development of an addictive personality.* Center City, MN: Hazelden.

Nietzsche, F. (1954). Thus spake Zarathustra. In W. Kaufman (Ed. & Trans.), *The portable Nietzsche* (pp. 103–439). New York, NY: Viking. (Original work published 1883)

Nietzsche, F. (1969). *On The Geneology of Morals and Ecce Homo,* Trans. Walter Kaufman and R. J. Hollingdale. New York: Vintage Books

Nixon, G. (2012). Transforming the addicted person's counterfeit quest for wholeness through three stages of recovery: A Wilber transpersonal spectrum of development clinical perspective. *International Journal of Mental Health Addiction, 10*(3), 407–427.

O'Brien, M. E. (1997). A serious problem comes out of the closet. *Post Graduate Medicine, 102,* 198–206.

Orford, J. (2000). *Excessive appetites: A psychological view of addiction* (2nd ed.). Chichester, England: Wiley.

Overton, W. F. (2007). A coherent metatheory for dynamic systems: Relational organicism-contextualism. *Human Development, 50,* 154–159.

Padaiga, Z., Subata, E., & Vanagas, G. (2007). Outpatient methadone maintenance treatment program quality of life and health of opioid-dependent persons in Lithuania. *Medicina (Kaunas), 43,* 235–241.

Parry, C. D. H., Pluddermann, A., & Myers, B. J. (2005). Heroin treatment demand in South Africa: Trends from two large metropolitan sites (January 1997-December 2003). *Drug and Alcohol Review, 24,* 419–423.

Pilgrim, D. (2002). The biopsychosocial model in Anglo-American psychiatry: Past, present, and future. *Journal of Mental Health, 11,* 585–594.

Polkinghorne, D. E. (2004). *Practice and the human sciences.* Albany, NY: SUNY Press.

Prentiss, C. (2005). *The alcoholism and addiction cure.* Malibu, CA: Power Press.

Proschaska, J. O., & DiClemente, C. C. (1992). Stages of change in the modification of problem behaviors. In M. Hersen, R. M. Eisler, & P. M. Miller (Eds.), *Progress in behavior modification, 28* (pp. 184–214). Sycamore, IL: Sycamore Press.

Ray, O., & Ksir, C. (2004). *Drugs, society, and human behavior.* New York, NY: McGraw-Hill.

Reber, J. S., & Osbeck, L. (2005). Social psychology: Key issues, assumptions and implications. In B. D. Slife, J. S. Reber, & F. C. Richardson (Eds.), *Critical thinking about psychology: Hidden assumptions and plausible alternatives* (pp. 63–79). Washington, DC: APA Books.

Richardson, F. C. (2002). Current dilemmas, hermeneutics, and power. *Journal of Theoretical and Philosophical Psychology. 22*, 114–132.

Richardson, F. C. (2005). Psychotherapy and modern dilemmas. In B. D. Slife, F. C. Richardson, & J. S. Reber (Eds.), *Critical thinking about psychology: Hidden assumptions and plausible alternatives* (pp. 17–38) . Washington, DC: American Psychological Association.

Ribes-Inesta, E. (2003). Concepts and theories: Relation to scientific categories. In K. A. Lattel & P. N. Chase (Eds.), *Behavior theory and philosophy*, (pp. 147–166). New York, NY: Kluwer Academic/Plenum.

Rioux, D. (1996). Shamanic healing techniques: Toward holistic addiction counseling. *Alcoholism Treatment Quarterly, 14*(1), 59–69.

Ritzer, G. (1991). Reflections on the rise of metatheorizing in sociology. *Sociological Perspectives, 34*(3), 237–248.

Roberts, A. J., & Koob, G. J. (1997). The neurobiology of addition: An overview. *Alcohol and Health Research World, 21*(2), 101–143.

Ronell, A. (1993). *Crack wars: Literature, addiction, mania*. Lincoln, NE: University of Nebraska Press.

Sartre, J. (1971). *Being and nothingness*. NewYork, NY: Bantam. (Original work published 1943)

Schuckit, M. A. (1980). A theory of alcohol and drug abuse: A genetic approach. In D. J. Lettieri, M. Sayers, & H. W. Persons (Eds.), *Theories on drug abuse: Selected contemporary perspectives* (NIDA Research Monograph No. 30; pp. 297–302). Rockville, MD: National Institute of Drug Abuse.

Schuckit, M. A., Goodwin, D. W., & Winokur, G. A. (1972). A long-term study of sons of alcoholics. *Alcohol Health and Research World, 19*, 172–175.

Siegel, R. (1984). The natural history of hallucinogens. In B. Jacobs (Ed.), *Hallucinogens: Neurochemical, behavioral, and clinical perspectives* (pp. 1–18). New York, NY: Raven Press.

Sremac, S. (2010). Addiction, narrative and spirituality: Theoretical-mythological approaches and overview. Retrieved 10 July 2010 from: http://www.academia.edu/327196/Addiction_Narrative_and_Spirituality_Theoretical-Methodological_Approaches_and_Overview

Shaffer, H. J. (1986). Conceptual crisis and the addictions: A philosophy of science perspective. *Journal of Substance Abuse Treatment, 3*, 285–296.

Shaffer, H. J. (1995). A clinical update on the addictions. In *workshop, The Addictions, March, Harvard Medical School, Boston*.

Shaffer, H. J. (1997).The most important unresolved issue in the addictions: Conceptual chaos. *Substance Use and Misuse, 32*, 1573–1580.

Shaffer, H. J., LaPlante, D. A., LaBrie, R. A., Kidman, R. C., Donato, A. N., & Stanton, M. V. (2004). Toward a syndrome model of addiction: Multiple expressions, common etiology. *Harvard Review of Psychiatry, 12*, 367–364.

Shealy, S. (2009). Toward an integrally informed approach to alcohol and drug treatment: Bridging the science and spirit gap. *Journal of Integral Theory and Practice, 4*(3), 109–126.

Shiffman, S., & Wills, T. A. (Eds.) (1985). *Coping and substance abuse.* New York, NY: Academic Press.

Shuttleworth, A. (2002). Turning towards a bio-psycho-social way of thinking. *European Journal of Psychotherapy, 5,* 205–223.

Skinner, Q. (1985). *The return of grand theory in the human sciences.* Cambridge, England: Cambridge University Press.

Slife, B. D. (2005). Taking practice seriously: Toward a relational ontology. *Journal of Theoretical and Philosophical Psychology, 24,* 157–178.

Slife, B. D., & Hopkins, R. (2005). Alternative assumptions for neuroscience: Formulating a true monism. In B. D. Slife, J. S. Reber, & F. C. Richardson (Eds.), *Critical thinking about psychology: Hidden assumptions and plausible alternatives* (pp. 121–147). Washington, DC: APA Books.

Slife, B. D., & Richardson, F. C. (2008). Problematic ontological underpinnings of positive psychology: A strong relational alternative. *Theory & Psychology, 18,* 699–723.

Smuts, J. C. (1926). *Holism and evolution.* London, England: MacMillan.

Solomon, L. J., & Corbit, J. (1974). An opponent-process theory of motivation: Temporal dynamics of affects. *Psychological Review, 81,* 119–145.

Taillefer, M. C., Dupuis, G., Roberge, M. A., & Le May, S. (2003). Health-related quality of life models: Systematic review of the literature. *Social Indicators Research, 64,* 293–323.

Temple, M., & Gall, T. L. (2016). Working through existential anxiety toward authenticity: A spiritual journey of meaning making. *Journal of Humanistic Psychology,* š1-26. doi:10.1177/0022167816629968

Thune, C. E. (1977). Alcholism and the archetypal past: A phenomenological perpserctive of Alchoholics Anonymous. *Quaterly Journal of Studies of Alchohol, 38*, 75–88.

Ulman, R. B., & Paul, H. (2006) *The self psychology of addiction and its treatment: Narcissus in wonderland.* New York, NY: Routledge.

Vaillant, G. E. (1995). *The natural history of alcoholism revisited.* Cambridge, MA: Harvard University Press.

Vanhooren, S., Leijssen, M., & Dezutter, J. (2017). Ten prisoners on a search for meaning: A qualitative study of loss and growth during incarceration. *The Humanistic Psychologist, 45*, 162–178

Volkow, N. D., Fowler, J. S., & Wang, G. J. (2002). Role of dopamine in drug reinforcement and addiction in humans: results from imaging studies. *Behavioral pharmacology, 13*, 355–366.

Wallace, J. (1985). Predicting the onset of compulsive drinking in alcoholics: A biopsychosocial model. *Alcohol, 2*, 589–595.

Wallace, J. (1993). Modern disease models of alcoholism and other chemical dependencies: The new biopsychosocial models. *Drugs and Society, 8*, 69–87.

Wallis, S. E. (2010). Toward a science of metatheory. *Integral Review, 6*(3), 73–115.

Walters, J. P. (2007). *Directors drug control strategy: Policy statement, October 2.* Washington, DC: Office of National Drug Control Policy.

Weil, A. (1972). *The natural mind.* Boston, MA: Houghton Mifflin.

West, R. (2005). *Theory of addiction.* Malden, MA: Blackwell.

White, W. (1996). *Pathways: From the culture of addiction to the culture of recovery.* Center City, MN: Hazelden.

White, W. (1998). *Slaying the dragon: The history of addiction Treatment and Recovery in America.* Bloomington, IL: Chestnut Health Systems.

Whitfield, C. L. (1991). *Co-dependence, healing the human condition.* Deerfield Beach, FL: Health Communications.

Wilber, K. (1995). *Sex, ecology, spirituality: The spirit of evolution.* Boston, MA: Shambhala.

Wilber, K. (2000). *Integral psychology: Consciousness, spirit, psychology, therapy.* Boston, MA: Shambhala.

Wilber, K. (2003a). Excerpt A: An integral age at the leading edge. Retrieved from http://www.kenwilber.com/Writings/PDF/ExcerptA_KOSMOS_2003.pdf

Wilber, K. (2003b). Excerpt B: The many ways we touch: Three principles helpful for any integrative approach. Retrieved from http://www.kenwilber.com/Writings/PDF/ExcerptB_KOSMOS_2003.pdf

Wilber, K. (2006). *Integral spirituality: A startling new role for religion in the modern and postmodern world.* Boston, MA: Integral Books.

Wills, T. A., & Shiffman, S. (1985). *Coping and substance use: A conceptual framework.* Orlando, FL: Academic Press.

Winkelman, M. (2001). Alternative and traditional medicine approaches for substance abuse programs: A shamanic perspective. *International Journal of Drug Policy, 12,* 337–351.

Wurmser, L. (1995). Compulsiveness and conflict: The distinction between description and explanation in the treatment of addictive behavior. In S. Dowling (Ed.), *The psychology and treatment of addictive behavior* (pp. 43–64). Madison, CT: International Universities Press.

Yalom, I. (1980). *Existential psychotherapy.* New York, NY: Basic Books.

Zoja, L. (1989). *Drugs, addiction and initiation: The modern search for ritual.* Boston, MA: Sigo.

ABOUT THE AUTHOR

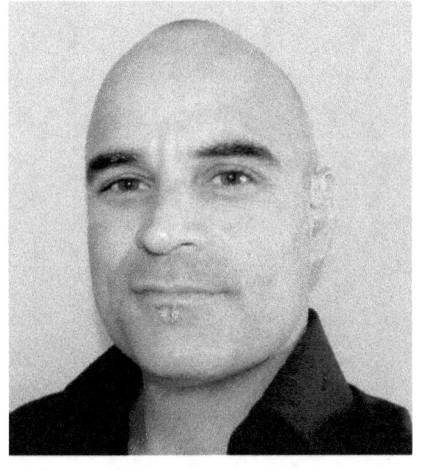

*G*uy du Plessis, MA, has a Master's degree in Psychology, and is a registered counselor at the Health Professions Council of South Africa. He is currently pursuing his PhD degree at the University of South Africa, and conducted doctoral research as a visiting scholar at the University of Leuven (KU Leuven). He has worked in the addiction treatment milieu for over 17 years as an addictions counselor, head of treatment, program & clinical director, trainer, and researcher. He is the author of *An Integral Guide to Recovery: Twelve Steps and Beyond*, and co-author of *Mind-Body Workbook for Addiction: Effective Tools for Relapse Prevention and Recovery*, and has published academic articles in the fields of addiction treatment and studies, theoretical psychology, and philosophy. He is on the faculty at the School of Behavioral Sciences at California Southern University, and faculty at the Wayne Institute for Advanced Psychotherapy at Bellarmine University, and the co-director of the Experiential-Existential Psychotherapy Research Center. He provides online therapy, training and consulting through his website at www.guyduplessis.com and can be contacted at guy@guyduplessis.com.

INDEX

SYMBOLS

(8PP). See eight primordial perspectives

A

A.A. See Alcoholics Anonymous
addiction
  brain disease 5, 74, 99
  etiological models xvi, xxiv, xxix, xxxii, 33, 46–47, 49–51, 55, 59, 61
addictionology xxv, 10, 25, 27, 29–30, 45, 50, 59, 128
alcohol xxiv, xxvii, 4, 7, 10, 13, 21–22, 29, 39–41, 75–76, 83, 86–87, 106, 113, 129, 132–139, 143, 144
Alcoholics Anonymous 15, 18–19, 86, 129, 138
alcoholism 4, 15–16, 20, 76, 112–113, 130–131, 136, 142, 145
Alexander, Bruce 1–3, 29
altered states of consciousness (ASCs) xxxii, 4, 13–14, 85, 139

AQAL
  Lines of Development 79
  Quadrants xv, 46, 52, 55, 72–73, 79, 87–88, 115, 135
  stages of development 58, 80–81, 84, 122
  states of consciousness xxxii, 4, 13–14, 85, 139
  Types xv, 87
ASCs. *See altered states of consciousness*
autopoiesis theory 10–11, 53, 55

B

basic existential needs 107, 110
being-in-recovery 125
being-in-the-world 63, 77, 96, 98–99, 106, 113, 115, 117–118
Binswanger, Ludwig 101
biology 37, 39–41, 45, 50, 75
biopsychosocial model vii–viii, xvi–xvii, xxxiii, 4, 24–25, 30, 32, 34, 36, 134, 138, 141, 145
  ontological abstractionism 34

ontological foundation xxvi, xxxiii,
    33, 59, 128
  prioritizing of factors 38
  separation of factors 37–38
Boss, Medard 45
BPS. *See biopsychosocial model*
Bugental, James 103
Burroughs, William 78

C
Califano, Joseph xxvii
cocaine 6, 90
compound models xxv–xxvi, xxxiii,
    27, 30–33, 42, 51, 59
compulsive behaviors 12
compulsive/excessive behavior models
    xxxii, 4, 12
conceptual chaos xxi, xxv, xxviii, xxxiii,
    27, 29, 33, 42, 43, 71, 128, 143
conceptual confusion 33, 42
conditioning/reinforcement behavioral
    models xxxii, 3, 10–11, 55
Cook-Greuter. *See Cook-Greuter,*
    Suzanne
Cook-Greuter, Suzanne 120
coping/social learning models xxxii,
    3, 9–10, 55
coping styles 88, 91
culture of addiction 78–79, 145
culture of recovery 145

D
Daseinsanalysis 97–98, 102
definitional confusion xxv, xxxiii, 30,
    127
Dewey, John 19, 132
disease model of addiction 5, 99

dislocation 30
doing-in-recovery 125
dopamine xxvii, 145
dukkha 114
Du Plessis, Guy i–iv, vii, xiii–xviii,
    xxiv–xxvi, xxviii, 2–3, 30, 46–48,
    54–55, 57, 64, 72–73, 80–82, 87,
    90–91, 96, 105, 115–117, 119,
    123–124, 132–133, 147
Dupuy, John xx, 84

E
Edwards, Mark xx
eight primordial perspectives 52
  autopoiesis theory 10–11, 53, 55
  empiricism 53, 55
  ethnomethodology 53
  hermeneutics 53, 55, 142
  phenomenology xvii, 53, 55, 97,
    100, 137
  social autopoiesis theory 53, 55
  structuralism 53, 55
  systems theory 53, 55
empiricism 53, 55
enactment xv, 48–52, 58–60, 63, 65,
    68, 70, 140
Engel, George 31
epistemic fallacies 67
epistemological pluralism 49, 57–58
epistemology xvi, xxviii, 32, 43, 48,
    57, 60, 63, 65, 98
Esbjörn-Hargens, Sean 48
ethnomethodology 55
etiological models of addiction
  biopsychosocial model vii–viii, xvi–
    xvii, xxxiii, 4, 24–25, 30, 32, 34,
    36, 134, 138, 141, 145

compulsive/excessive behavior
models xxxii, 4, 12
conditioning/reinforcement
behavioral models xxxii, 3,
10–11, 55
coping/social learning models
xxxii, 3, 9–10, 55
existential/spiritual and altered
states of consciousness models 13
genetic/physiological models xxxii,
3–5, 55–56
personality/intrapsychic models
xxxii, 3, 7, 56
social/environmental models xxxii,
3, 6–7
transtheoretical model xxxiii, 4, 25,
55, 80, 132
twelve step programs xxxii, 4, 15,
18, 20, 22, 77, 111
existential 140
existential anxiety 99, 103–104, 144
existential foundation 42, 96–97, 130
existentialism 100
existential phenomenology 97, 100
existential philosophy 97, 99–101,
106, 113–114
existential psychology 97, 101–102
existential/spiritual and altered states
of consciousness models 13
existential therapy 97, 101–103

F
Flores, Philip xx
Forman, Mark xxvii
freedom ix, 95, 102–106, 108, 114,
139
Freud, Sigmund 22, 98

G
Gardner, Howard 80
genetic/physiological models xxxii,
3–5, 55–56
genetics 4, 36, 74
Gianotti, Patricia iv, xx
Gorman, Adam iv, xx

H
Hazard, Rowland 16
Heidegger, Martin 99
hermeneutics 53, 55, 142
heroin 3, 6, 78, 90, 131, 141
high-altitude stage recovery 82, 84
higher power 19, 77
holism xvi, 64, 105, 144
holistic approaches xxviii
horizontal development 121, 124
Husserl, Edmund 100, 136

I
IEP. *See integral methodological pluralism*
IMP. *See integral epistemological pluralism*
ineffectiveness of treatment xvi, xxv,
30, 127
ineffectual treatment 27, 41–43
integral enactment theory 48–49, 58,
63, 68, 70
integral epistemological pluralism 49, 57
integral metatheory i, xviii, xxviii,
xxxi–xxxii, 45, 133
integral meta-therapy xxviii, xxxiii,
72, 91, 93, 95
integral methodological pluralism 49,
52–53, 132, 138

integral ontological pluralism 49, 60
integral pluralism 48–50, 57–58, 63, 69, 133
integral theory i, iv, xv–xvi, xxvi–xxviii, xxxii–xxxiii, 43, 46–49, 54–55, 58–59, 63–70, 72, 79–82, 91–93, 96–97, 115, 128, 132–134, 138, 140, 144
   critique iii, xvi, xx, xxxiii, 15, 18–19, 25, 27, 30, 37, 42, 45, 48, 65–71, 96, 140
   Wilber, Ken ii, xv, xx, xxv, xxviii, xxxi–xxxii, 19–20, 46–47, 49–50, 52–55, 57–58, 64, 67–69, 72, 80, 83, 85, 92, 121, 146
Integral Transformative Practices 92
integrated recovery meta-therapy xvii, xxi, xxxiii, 93, 95
   existential foundation 96–97
   integral foundation xvi, xxviii, xxxiii, 91
   integrated recovery graph 120, 122
   integrated recovery program iii, 96, 117–120
   integrated recovery wheel xvii, 118, 122–123
   monthly integrated recovery index 124
   recovery dimensions iv, 115–118, 120, 122–124
   weekly integrated recovery index 124
integrated recovery model 117, 132
interpersonal relationships 22
IOP. *See integral ontological pluralism*
IRMt. *See integrated recovery meta-therapy*
ITP. *See integral transformative practices*

J
James, William 17–18, 76
Jaspers, Karl 101
Jung, Carl 13, 16–18, 30, 72, 76, 137

K
Kierkegaard, Søren 99–100, 113, 137
Kohut, Heinz 7–8, 20–21, 23, 78–79, 89, 91, 137
Kuhn, Thomas 20, 49

L
Laing, R.D. 102
legitimation crisis xxv
lens-field 63, 65
libidinal autonomy 22
lines of development 79–80
logotherapy 77, 101–102

M
masculine types 90
materialism 50
Max-Neef, Alfred 107–109, 115, 122, 139
May, Rollo 101, 103
metaparadigmatic xxvi, xxxii, 26, 48, 53, 56, 92–93
meta-reality xxxi
metatheoretical framework ii, xvii, xxviii, xxxii, 26, 96
metatheorising xxix, xxxi, 66
metatheory i, xv, xvii–xviii, xxviii–xxxii, 26, 45–46, 48, 66–67, 70, 133, 139, 141, 145
methamphetamine 6, 90
methodological pluralism 49, 52–53, 57, 63, 132, 138, 140

methodology xvi, xxviii, xxxii, 2, 15, 43, 49, 51, 56, 58, 60, 62, 65, 91, 96, 97–98
mindfulness 96
modes of being-in-recovery 125
multiparadigm research xxxii
Murray, Tom 51, 58, 67–70, 140

N

narcissism 9, 20, 23–24, 118, 137
neurobiology 4–5, 38–39, 142
neurophysiology 55, 74
Nietzsche, Friedrich 71, 99, 141
Nixon, Gary 47–48, 83–84, 141

O

object hunger 21, 22
ontological abstractionism 34, 35
ontological depth xxix, 63
ontological foundation xxvi, xxxiii, 32–34, 37, 42, 59, 128
ontological pluralism xxix, 49, 51, 57–60, 68–69
ontological relationality 34–35
ontological span xxix, 52, 58, 63
ontology
  ontological abstractionism 34–35
  ontological pluralism xxix, 49, 51, 57–60, 68–69
  ontological relationality 34, 35
  ontological span xxix, 52, 58, 63

P

Paul, Harry 76
Pavlovian conditioning 11, 136
personality/intrapsychic models xxxii, 3, 7, 55–56

phenomenology xvii, 53, 55, 97, 100, 137
positivism 50
proto-integral thinker 64

Q

quadrants
  lower-left quadrant 78
  lower-right quadrant 79
  upper-left quadrant 75, 80
  upper-right quadrant 73

R

Rank, Otto 101
recovery
  recovery program iii, 77, 80, 96, 110, 117–121, 124–126
  Twelve Step xxxii, 4, 15–20, 22–23, 51, 73, 77, 79, 83–84, 96, 111, 129, 133, 147
recovery dimensions
  environmental 6, 115, 118
  existential iv, xvi–xvii, 4, 13, 15, 42, 50–51, 75, 77, 82–83, 96–111, 113–115, 118, 125–126, 130, 132, 140, 144, 146, 148
  intellectual iii, 115, 118, 138
  physical 115, 118
  psychological iii, xxvii, 7, 9–10, 12, 14, 24–25, 31, 37, 74, 78, 82, 89, 115, 118, 129–131, 135–136, 141, 147
  social 115, 118
recovery-in-the-world 96, 115
recovery stages
  early stage 82–83
  high altitude stage 81

middle stage 83
Nixon, Gary 47–48, 83–84, 141
transpersonal stage 83–84
reinforcement models 11
relapse prevention iii, 82, 84, 138, 147
reward deficiency syndrome 62, 86, 98, 130

S
Sartre, Jean-Paul 99, 114, 143
satisfiers
    inhibiting satisfiers 109
    pseudo-satisfiers 109, 122
    singular satisfiers 109–110
    synergic satisfiers 109
    violators or destroyers 109–110
Schneider, Kirk 103
self-contained individualities 37
self-medication hypothesis 8, 78
self-object
    idealized self-object 21, 118
    mirroring self-object 21, 89
    object hunger 21–22
    self-object responsiveness 8, 20, 22
    transitional object 23
self psychology 20, 106, 145
self psychology perspective of twelve step programs 20
serotonin xxvii, 39–40
Silkworth, William D. 17–18
single-factor models 24–25, 30–31, 56, 61
Smuts, Jan
    fields 64–65
    holism xvi, 64, 105
    Holism and Evolution 64, 105
    lens-field 63, 65
social autopoiesis theory 53, 55
social/environmental models xxxii, 3, 6–7
social learning xxxii, 3, 9–12, 24, 55, 129
spectator knowledge 19
spirituality 13, 77, 130, 134, 138, 143, 146
structuralism 53, 55
systems theory 55

T
Thatcher, Ebby 16–17
theory of human scale development 107–108, 115
therapy xvii, xxi, xxviii, xxxiii, 72, 81, 84, 91, 93, 95–97, 101–103, 111, 120, 132, 134, 137, 139, 146, 148
third-order ontology 61, 62
transference disorders 23
transtheoretical model xxxiii, 4, 25, 55, 80, 132
trauma 74, 76, 130
Twelve Step programs
    critique of twelve step programs 18
    history of AA and the twelve steps 16
typology
    feminine 90–91
    masculine 90–91
    types xxix, xxxii, 5, 23, 32, 46, 72, 80, 85, 87, 88, 90, 107, 109, 120, 135

U
Ulman, Richard 7–9, 76, 89–90, 106, 145

V

van Deurzen, Emmy 102
vertical development 120–122, 124

W

Weathers, Robert iii, xx, 84
weekly integrated recovery index 124
West, Robert xxv, 2–3, 5, 8, 26, 61, 145
White, William xxv, 13, 29–30, 35, 41–42, 46, 78, 127–128, 138, 145
Wilber, Ken
  AQAL xv, xxxi, 46, 48, 52, 70, 72, 133, 135, 140
  integral theory i, iv, xv–xvi, xxvi, xxviii, xxxii–xxxiii, 43, 46–49, 54, 58, 63–70, 72, 79–80, 82, 91–93, 96–97, 115, 128, 134, 140
Wilson, Bill 13, 16–18, 76

Y

Yalom, Irwin 16, 101–104, 146

Z

Zoja, Luigi 1, 14, 77, 146

www.ingramcontent.com/pod-product-compliance
Lightning Source LLC
Chambersburg PA
CBHW070825250426
43671CB00036B/2081